1902-2002

ONE HUNDRED YEARS *of* MEDICINE

|

WAKE FOREST UNIVERSITY

ONE HUNDRED YEARS
of MEDICINE

❧

*The Legacy of Yesterday,
the Promise of Tomorrow*

❧

Donna S. Garrison

EDITOR

WAKE FOREST UNIVERSITY HEALTH SCIENCES PRESS

WINSTON-SALEM

NORTH CAROLINA

Design by Biomedical Communications

Printed in the United States of America

ISBN: 0-9644070-6-X

Contents

The Legacy of Yesterday, the Promise of Tomorrow

Through pictures of people, places, and events dating from 1902 in Wake Forest, North Carolina, to 2002 in Winston-Salem, this book commemorates and honors the first 100 years of medicine at Wake Forest University.

The evolution of the Wake Forest University School of Medicine is a wonderful story. In 1902, thirteen students began a two-year course in medicine as part of the undergraduate curriculum at Wake Forest College. At the time of this publication, 424 students attend a four-year medical school that receives national recognition for its innovation in medical education, research, and patient care. Although The North Carolina Baptist Hospitals, Incorporated, is an institution separate from the School of Medicine, the histories and activities of the hospital and school intertwine inextricably to form the Wake Forest University Baptist Medical Center. Like the staff of Aesculapius, with its serpent encircling the rod to form the symbol associated with the medical profession, it is difficult to determine where the school ends and the hospital begins. In this book, pictures of both institutions help to tell the story of the School of Medicine.

For this project a committee of eleven people reviewed yearbooks from 1902 to 2002, thousands of photographs housed in the Dorothy Carpenter Medical Archives, and hundreds of additional pictures stored electronically and in slide files in the Department of

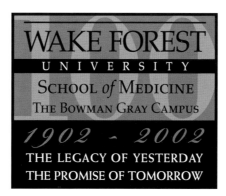

WAKE FOREST
UNIVERSITY
SCHOOL of MEDICINE
THE BOWMAN GRAY CAMPUS
1902 – 2002
THE LEGACY OF YESTERDAY
THE PROMISE OF TOMORROW

Biomedical Communications. The committee devoted considerable effort to the identification of the people, buildings, and events central to the first 100 years of Wake Forest University School of Medicine. Still, some important parts of the story are missing. Numerous individuals who have contributed significantly to the development and progress of the School of Medicine do not appear because photographs were unavailable, because space was limited, or because of inadvertent oversights during the selection process.

Special thanks go to those directly involved with the creation of this book: Doug Maynard for his vision; Katherine Davis for her invaluable knowledge of history and her identification of people, places, and events; Linda Bell and Tammy Ball for the design of the book; Donna Garrison for writing the narrative; Dianne Johnson for her assistance during the review of material stored in the Archives; Vicki Johnson for organizing the photographs into appropriate categories; Mike Sprinkle for his time and energy in helping to select photographs and identify subjects; Parks Welch for his help and the dedication of his staff to the project; and Frank James, whose leadership and tireless efforts in organizing the group made this book possible.

The Legacy of Yesterday . . .

The Wake Forest Era and the Two-Year School

For the institution now known as Wake Forest University School of Medicine, history began on the campus of Wake Forest Institute. Incorporated in the winter of 1833, the Institute began regular operations in February 1834 in the community of Wake Forest, located in Wake County near North Carolina's capital city of Raleigh. During its first five years of operation, the Institute enrolled an average of 89 students per year. It was chartered in 1838 as Wake Forest College, and according to the charter, the mission of the institution was to provide "an education, both physical, intellectual and moral" that would encourage "the formation of character" and would prepare its students for "honor, usefulness, and happiness." Wake Forest operated as a college of liberal arts from its beginnings until 1894, when the School of Law was established.

As early as 1849, a "Medical Department" had been proposed. The absence of medical colleges in North Carolina and the resulting necessity of sending students (and their dollars) north to pursue a medical education were widely deplored. The proximity of Wake Forest to Raleigh made its location attractive for development of a medical school, but eventually the economic hardships brought about by the Civil War sidelined this project before it began. Although the idea of a medical "diploma mill" was tempting to some as a way to increase capital, this approach was rejected and plans were tabled for 20 years. While no definitive progress toward establishment of a medical school was evident, by the academic year 1886-1887 the college's catalogue included a new program: a "Course Preliminary to the Study of Medicine," intended as a remedy for the "want of proper preliminary training" of medical students at many medical colleges. The full course of study included physics, chemistry, physiology, botany, mathematics, and Latin.

Dr. C. E. Taylor, president of Wake Forest College, persisted in his pursuit of a medical school for his institution, and his perseverance ultimately was rewarded when the two-year Wake Forest College Medical School was established in 1902. According to Coy C. Carpenter, M.D., who would later become dean of the medical school, "Dr. Taylor's genius lay in getting tasks done without controversy, and in his characteristic manner he quietly succeeded in establishing a school of law and a school of medicine." He insisted that the academic standards of the school be maintained at the highest possible level and that it produce graduates who would improve the lives, not only of North Carolinians, but of Southerners in general. He firmly believed, however, that Wake Forest Medical School should offer only a two-year program, as "only an institution which can offer the advantage of great hospitals and extensive clinical opportunities of a large city is in a position" to confer a medical degree.

The first dean of the medical school was Dr. Fred K. Cooke (1902-1905), and the first class enrolled 13 students. However, despite the best efforts of Drs. Cooke and Taylor, the beginnings of this medical venture were somewhat inauspicious, as seven of the original 13 failed their first year of course work.

The high standards upheld by the college president and the first medical dean were evident when, merely two years after the program was established, the Association of American Medical Colleges accepted Wake Forest College Medical School into membership in 1904. Unfortunately, Dr. Cooke found it necessary to resign the deanship in 1905 because poor health prevented him from devoting his full attention to the school. He went back into private practice, but by 1910 Cooke was dead of a peptic ulcer. He was only 34 years old.

Cooke's successor, pathologist Watson S. Rankin, was a University of Maryland graduate who also studied at Johns Hopkins. He had joined the Wake Forest medical faculty in 1903, and as dean during the period 1905-1909 he insisted that training good doctors was the medical school's only reason for being and that the only way to accomplish that mission was to demand excellence from everyone involved. Although this position may seem unremarkable today, the fact is that a dozen medical schools existed at that time in North Carolina alone, and in 1910 Wake Forest's medical school was one of only 11 in the entire United States – a total of 160 schools – that required two years of college for admission.

The Flexner Report of 1910, a survey of medical education in the U.S. commissioned by the Carnegie Foundation for the Advancement of Teaching, included this in its Wake Forest report: "The laboratories of this little school are, as far as they go, models in their way. Everything about them indicates intelligence and earnestness." Rankin, whose accomplishments are reflected in the report, resigned in 1909 to become North Carolina's first Board of Health secretary. He continued to support the school as a trustee of the college and brought recognition to the medical school through his scientific studies on hookworm, the publication of which was instrumental in the elimination of the disease in the South.

When Rankin stepped down, John B. Powers, Jr., stepped up as acting dean for the 1909-1910 year and was appointed dean for 1910-1911. The young doctor's tenure was brief, however, as conflicts among the medical faculty led the trustees to terminate the position of dean in 1911. For most of a decade, individual medical faculty members reported directly to the president of Wake Forest College. This unsettled period at the Wake Forest Medical School paralleled a tumultuous time for medical education nationwide, during which a large number of medical schools folded, including many four-year schools. Of the 160 medical colleges in existence in 1907, only 100 remained in 1914. The survival of the medical program at Wake Forest is most likely the result, first, of its unwavering high standards and, second, its association with a highly respected liberal arts college.

The rapid turnover in administration during the school's first decade, though readily explained, contrasts sharply with the stability that has characterized its leadership since then. In 1919 the medical school had a new dean, its fourth in 17 years, and Thurman D. Kitchin would serve in that role until 1936. A general practitioner educated at Wake Forest College and Jefferson Medical College, Kitchin had joined the medical faculty in 1917. Under his watch the medical school moved to a fine new facility, the William Amos Johnson Medical Building, in 1933. Named for an anatomy instructor who taught for only one year before being killed in an automobile accident, the new building was a vast improvement over the cramped quarters of the Alumni Building, a portion of which had hosted the medical classes since 1905. In 1930 Kitchin took on the responsibility of the college presidency in addition to that of medical school dean. Under his leadership the medical school weathered the Great Depression as well as constant threats to its own existence and that of other two-year schools. Although he continued as president of Wake Forest College until 1950, Kitchin relinquished the role of dean to Coy C. Carpenter in 1936.

Coy Cornelius Carpenter was a 1922 graduate of the two-year Wake Forest College Medical School and of Syracuse University School of Medicine. He was appointed professor of pathology and physical diagnosis at Wake Forest in 1926 and in subsequent years became a close acquaintance and admirer of Dr. Kitchin. When Carpenter became dean in 1936, he was embarking on a quarter century of visionary leadership under which the school would be thoroughly transformed — in its structure, its location, and its identity.

◀ **Board of Trustees of Wake Forest College, in 1903**

Wake Forest College lists medicine as one of its "independent schools" in this 1903 announcement.
▼

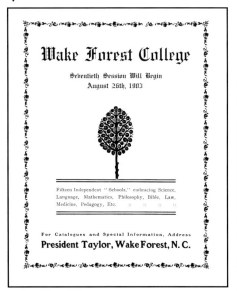

Entire faculty of Wake Forest College in 1903, including Fred K. Cooke, first dean of the medical school (1902-1905), bottom row, second from left; Watson S. Rankin, Cooke's successor as dean (1905-1909), far right, third down; and C. E. Taylor, president of Wake Forest College (1875-1905), far left, third down
▼

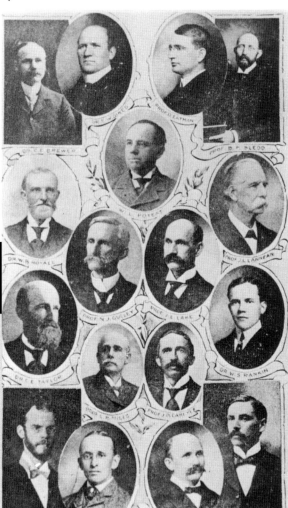

1902

1902 — *Two-year Wake Forest College Medical School opens—13 students enroll. Plans are made to establish four-year program*

1903 — *The Wright Brothers achieve first sustained aircraft flight at Kitty Hawk, North Carolina. Longest flight is one minute, 12 seconds*

1903 — *First surgical suture of a heart wound performed by Luther Hill*

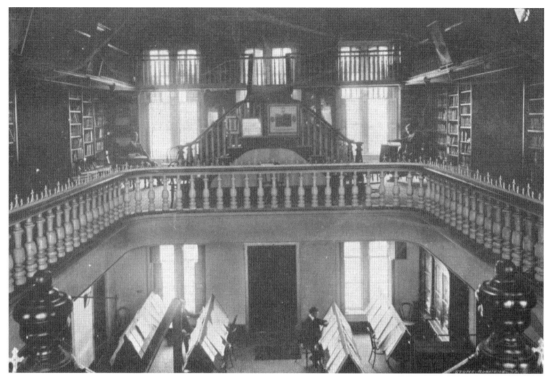

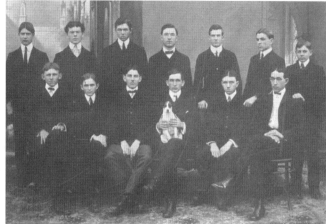

▲ The entering 1902 medical class, consisting of 13 students and, presumably, one mascot

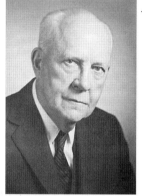

◄ Watson S. Rankin, pathologist and dean of the medical school (1905-1909), after Fred K. Cooke's resignation. Rankin himself resigned in 1909 to become the first secretary of the North Carolina Board of Health.

▲ The Wake Forest College library occupied the central hall of the Heck-Williams Building, with stacks on the upper level and a reading room on the first floor.

MEDICAL CLASS.

OFFICERS.

JOHN ARCHIBALD MCMILLAN,
PRESIDENT.

JOHN LAMBE PRITCHARD,
VICE-PRESIDENT.

ISAAC ARCHER HORNE,
SECRETARY AND TREASURER.

JOHN BREWER POWERS, JR.,
HISTORIAN.

MEMBERS.

NAME.	SOCIETY.	HOME ADDRESS.
PAUL CLENTON BRITTLE	ϒ	Menola, North Carolina
PAUL CRUMPLER	Φ	Clinton, North Carolina
THOMAS JOSEPH DEAN	ϒ	Cedar Rock, North Carolina
GEORGE NORFLEET HARRELL	ϒ	Potecasi, North Carolina
WILLIAM ALDEN HOGGARD	ϒ	Windsor, North Carolina
ISAAC ARCHER HORNE	ϒ	Pendleton, North Carolina
R. R. LUCAS	Φ	Plymouth, North Carolina
GEORGE A. MCLEMORE	Φ	Parkersburg, North Carolina
JOHN ARCHIBALD MCMILLAN	Φ	Riverton, North Carolina
PAUL HAYNE MITCHELL	ϒ	Ahoskie, North Carolina
HODGE ALBERT NEWELL	ϒ	Mapleville, North Carolina
JOHN BREWER POWERS, JR	Φ	Wake Forest, North Carolina
JOHN LAMBE PRITCHARD	ϒ	Burden, North Carolina
HOUSTON WINGATE VERNON	ϒ	Wake Forest, North Carolina

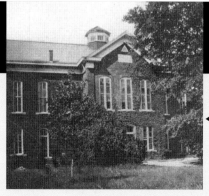

◄ One of the early buildings on the old Wake Forest College campus near Raleigh, in 1903

1903 — Radioactivity discovered and isolated by Pierre and Marie Curie of France

1904 — Construction of Panama Canal begins

1905

◄ Roster of officers and members of the 1903 medical class. John Brewer Powers, Jr., served briefly as dean of the medical school (1910-1911).

MEDICAL CLASS

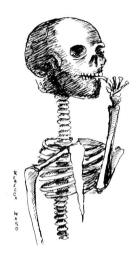

Officers

WINGATE M. JOHNSON, President.

RICHARD E. TIMBERLAKE, Vice-President.

HAL P. HARRIS, Secretary.

JOHN E. RAY, Treasurer.

ROBERT H. FREEMAN, Historian.

E. L. MORGAN, Poet.

◄ Medical class officers in 1906 included class president Wingate M. Johnson, who later became professor of clinical medicine and was Board of Trustees president. The rather grim art work is attributed to Rebecca Ward.

Gymnasium on old Wake Forest campus housed the original anatomy lab in the basement.
▼

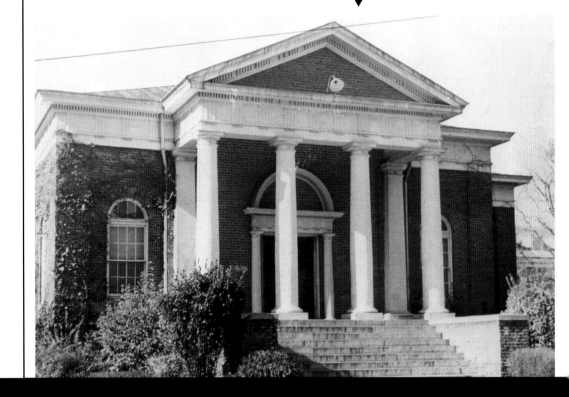

1905

1905 — Albert Einstein
introduces his
Theory of Relativity

1906 — Novocain
introduced by Einhorn

1906 — First successful
cornea transplant is accomplished
by Edouard Zirm

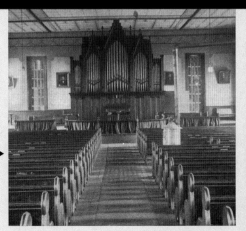

Interior of the Wake Forest ►
College chapel, in 1908.

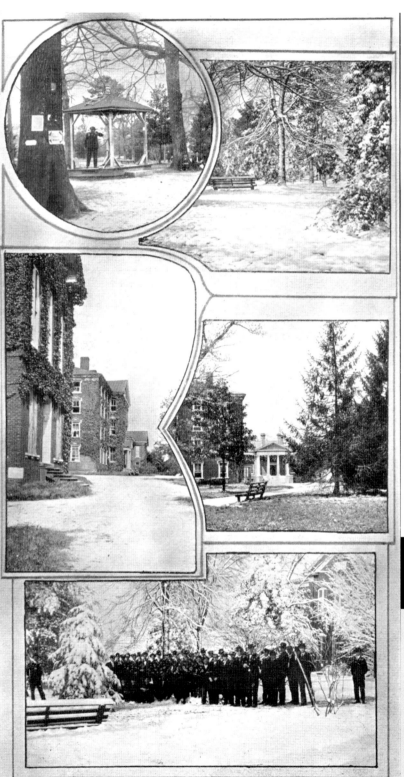

◀ Campus scenes from the 1908
Howler, the college yearbook

Medical Class Poem

❦ ❦ ❦

The Med. Students we do be,
And in time hope to see,
Some glad Commencement morn,
Another title our name adorn.
Our daily fare are stiffs and bones,
Served to the music (?) of Lectures tones.
Pills we'll roll and plasters make,
Now and then a bottle shake
To cure you we will honestly try—
And hope the bill to get, "by and by."

◀ Class poet was an important
office, for reasons not entirely
clear from this 1908 effort by
C. L. McCullers (see Medical
Class Officers, below).

1908 Medical Class Officers
▼

**"Doctor" Tom Jeffries,
greatly admired diener
who worked at Wake
Forest College from 1884
until four weeks before his
death on July 4, 1927. His
record for the longest
continuous service to the
school merited a bronze
bust, placed near the Lea
Chemistry Laboratory
shortly after his death.**
▼

Medical Class Officers

❦ ❦ ❦

C. M. PHIFER.................................President.
R. F. ELVINGTON.......................Vice-President.
B. S. BAZEMORE.............................Prophet.
C. L. McCULLERS.............................Poet.
CARL BELL ....Treasurer.
B. F. BUTLER...............................Secretary.
H. S. GEIGER...........................Chief Surgeon.

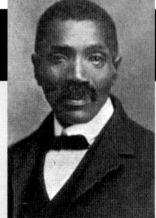

1908

*1906 — First tax-supported
library in North Carolina is
established in Winston-Salem*

*1906 — First fetal
electrocardiogram*

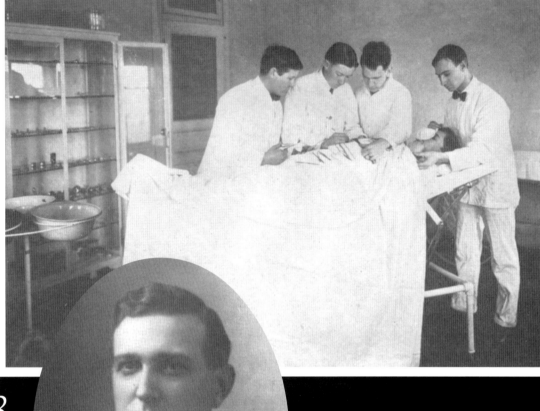

◀ Future physicians examine a patient anesthetized by inhaling ether, in 1908 before the introduction of intravenous anesthetics.

1911 Class Poem offers an interesting perspective on the healing art.

▼

The Med's Philosophy

PATIENT

"Oh, Mister Doctor, you're always in a dash
To make a new mortal of mangled up hash,
Or heal the wounds of a terrifying clash;
To cure the sick with your pills and bitter stuff,
Or keep giving it just to act the bluff;
Then smiling, tell us, 'you've only half enough.'
We'd rather die in excruciating pain,
And know exactly the one to blame,
Than breathe our last in your secret shame."

DOCTOR

"There's no risk in trusting us,
Yet you keep a cussing us.
Those we kill are out of the way—
Those we cure are those who pay."

POET.

1908

William ▶ Walton Kitchin in 1908, one of eight Kitchin brothers from Scotland Neck to attend Wake Forest College and father of W. W. Kitchin '38, Medical Alumni Association president in 1966.

1908 — Henry Ford produces the first Model T

Class officers in ▶ 1910. Class poet Luther T. Buchanan would chair the Department of Pathology and Bacteriology from 1917 until 1920.

Medical Class Officers

R. F. ELVINGTON	.	.	President
MIKE ROBERSON	.	.	Vice-President
W. M. WILLIS	.	.	Secretary
B. L. JONES	.	.	Treasurer
F. F. COX	.	.	Surgeon
P. P. GREEN	.	.	Historian
C. I. ALLEN	.	.	Prophet
LUTHER BUCHANAN	.	.	Poet

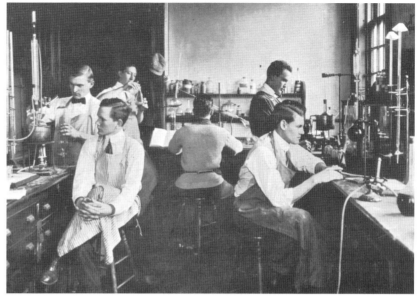

▲ Chemistry lab in 1911 required intense concentration and Hazmat aprons.

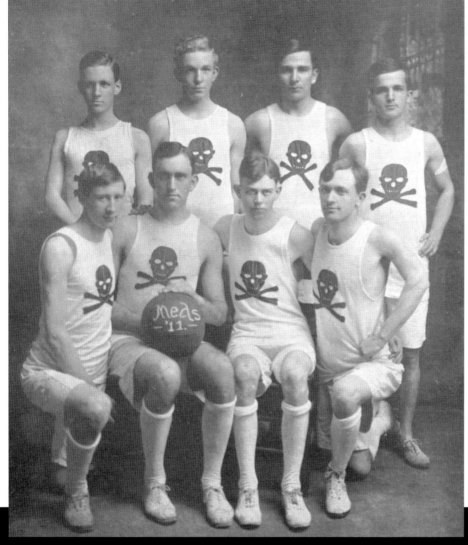

◄ ACC or no ACC, the Wake Forest "Meds" – and their uniforms – were formidable in 1911.

◄ The Alumni Building, built between 1904 and 1906, housed the medical school on the top floor, part of the second floor, and a portion of the basement until 1933.

1911

1908 — *Beginning of Prohibition*

1909 — *After many setbacks, Admiral Peary becomes first explorer to reach North Pole*

1909 — *Modern age of anesthesia begins as ether and chloroform are used as intravenous anesthetics*

1910 — *Leeches used to prevent clotting of blood in artificial kidneys*

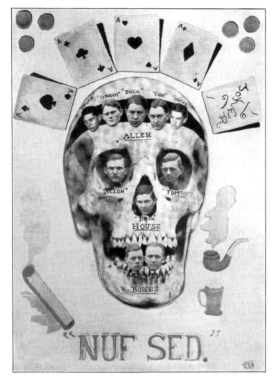

▲ Nuf sed? Maybe not (from the 1911 *Howler*)

"Gentlemen, synchronize your microscopes." ▶
Medical students hard at work in 1911.

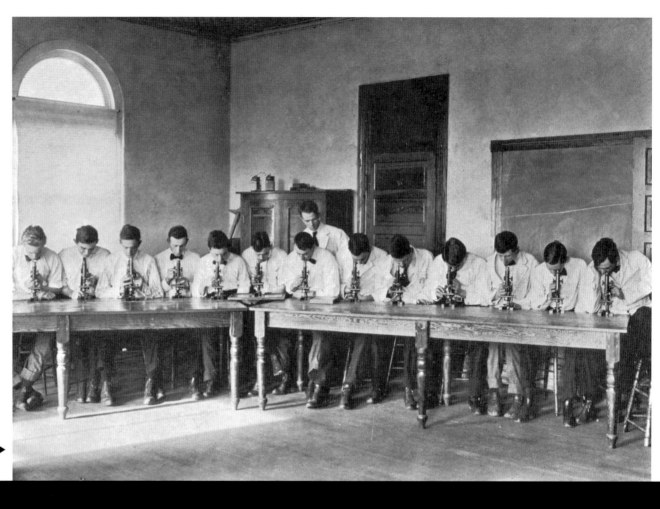

1911

1911 — Roland Anundsen
first to reach South Pole

1911 — US explorer Kiram Bingham
discovers lost Incan city of Machu Picchu

1912 — US Public Health
Service created

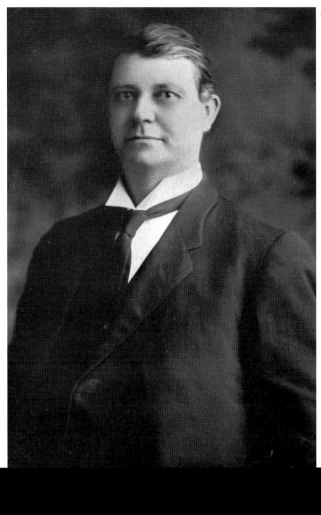

◀ **1912 photograph of Claude Kitchin, brother of William Walton Kitchin, graduate of Wake Forest Law School and later a U.S. Congressman**

LEVY L. CARPENTER, B.A., PHI.
Wake County, North Carolina

"For he who is honest is nobler,
Whatever his fortunes or birth."

Carpenter was once an agent for Students' Bibles and made a success in that arduous enterprise. This experience has stood him in good stead during his college career. He has always been a regular contributor to college publications, an excellent student, a wide reader; he expects to add the thorough preparation at the Seminary for a large field of usefulness. He has shown himself worthy of his honors by the faithful discharge of those duties conferred upon him. His quiet bearing and dignified demeanor will make him a fit minister to the needy. His democratic spirit, too, will assist him in his work. Levy does not cling entirely to the old idea, for he is open minded to see what is good and true; best of all, he is kind and sympathetic. May fortune ever assist this worthy pilgrim along the pathway of life.

Age 21, height 5 feet 7 inches, weight 137.

Associate Editor of THE HOWLER, '12; Editor in Chief of *The Student*, '12–'13; Senior Speaker '13; Historian of Senior Class, '13; Commencement Speaker, '13.

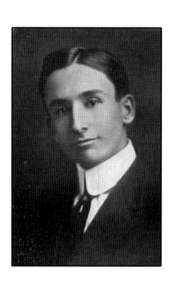

◀ **1913 photograph of Levy L. Carpenter, Baptist minister, editor of the *Biblical Recorder*, Wake Forest College graduate, and brother of Coy C. Carpenter**

1913

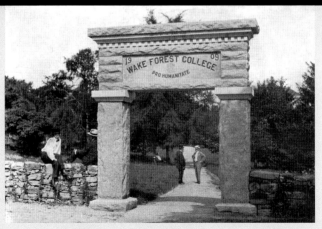

◀ **The Wake Forest College motto, *Pro Humanitate*, is visible on the entrance archway, built in 1909 by Coopers Monuments of Raleigh.**

1913 — Complete records of all births and deaths in North Carolina are begun

1913 — American College of Surgeons incorporated

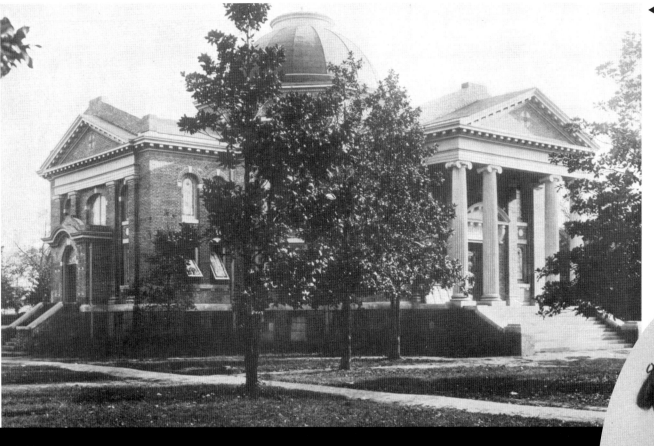

◀ Wake Forest Baptist
Church in 1916, two years
after its completion at a
cost of approximately
$50,000, on the south side
of the old campus

Unidentified class sponsor,
featured in the 1916 yearbook
▼

1914

1914 — Archduke Francis Ferdinand of
Austria is assassinated in Serbia,
leading to the start of
World War I

1914 — Income tax
becomes a federal law

By 1916 more than 30 ▶
students were enrolled in
the well-established
medical school.

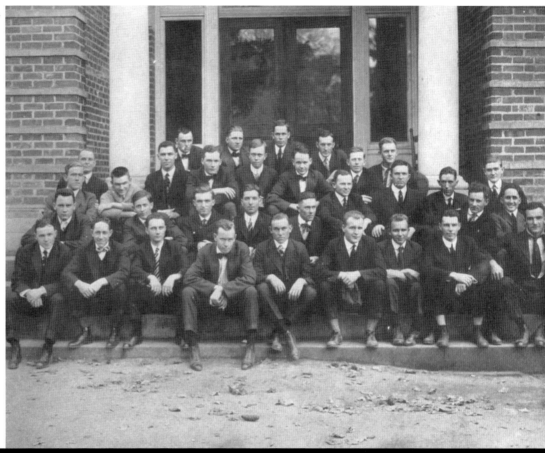

Wake Forest College Hospital. The facility opened as the
student infirmary in 1906 and contained several patient
rooms, an operating room, and a ward for patients with
contagious diseases, all built and equipped for $7,500.
The patient-day cost was approximately $1.75.
▼

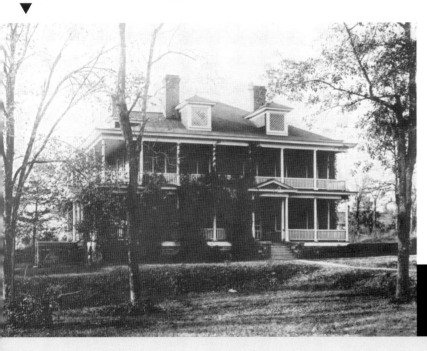

1916

1914 — Large-scale pasteurization of milk begins	1915 — Long distance telephone service begins between New York and San Francisco	1916 — A woman is elected to Congress for the first time	1916 — President Woodrow Wilson narrowly wins re-election with the campaign slogan "He kept us out of war"

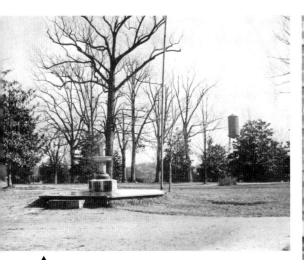

▲
The fountain on the old campus
as it appeared in 1918

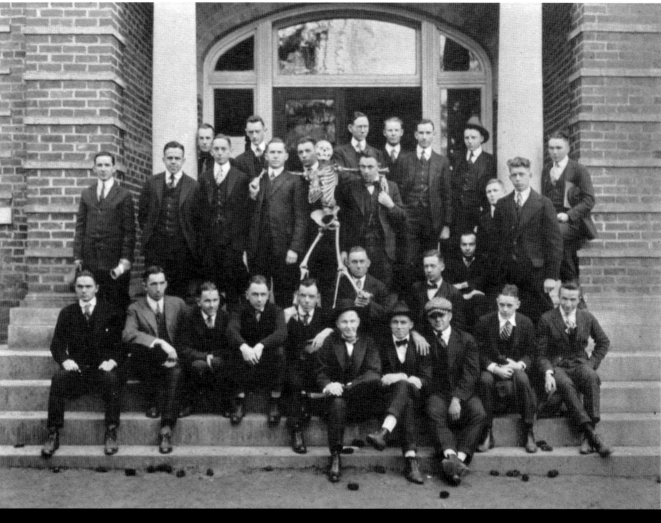

The 1918 medical class poses ▶
with unidentified companion
(second row, center).

1917

*1917 — Lenin leads Bolshevik
revolt after Romanovs abdicate*

*1917 — Bohr's Theory of
Atomic Structure
is introduced*

*1917 — Stethoscope designed
by David Sweeny Hills*

*1918 — Influenza epidemic
spreads, killing 70 million
worldwide and 500,000
Americans*

MEDICAL CLASS POEM

To write a poem, 'bout the Meds,
I have no inclination,
But they are here, a solemn fact,
To bless the whole creation.

Then let man rave, and rashly curse,
The men of vain professions,
For we will heal the world—that's us,
Of all its black digressions.

Some may take law and loudly shout,
To heal a nation's morals;
If they can't cure, they'll hurry out—
They long for showy laurels.

And others preach the Blessed Word,
About a loving Savior;
They often sneer—at least some do—
Because of man's behavior.

But be they good, or be they bad,
We're all put here to bless them;
A poor, disgraced, forsaken lad,
We'll do our best to heal him.

And as we go to fields unknown,
To Maines or Coloradoes,
We'll always share our healing balms
In day or in night's shadows.

So here we are, the good, the bad,
The brilliant and the stupid.
And most of us are mighty glad,
We're not a prey to Cupid.

For when at night, the cold winds blow,
We study books incessant.
Of man's chief ailments we must know,
And books make them translucent.

A – nat – o – my, His – tol – o – gy,
And various other subjects,
And bones, and cells, and forms, you see
We have to be their critics.

The smell of drugs is wondrous sweet
As lilacs on black boulders.
And out in life, the Meds you'll meet
Bear mankind on their shoulders.

—*Poet.*

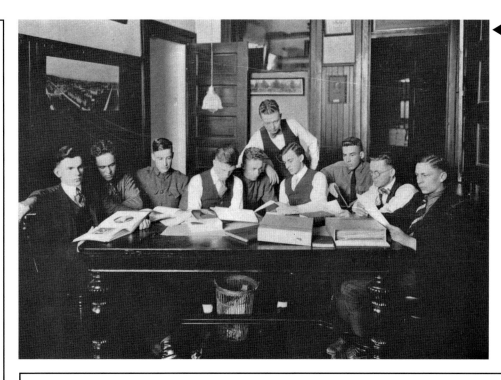

◀ **Studying for finals required a group effort in 1919.**

MEDICAL CLASS OFFICERS

J. L. SOWERS, President	C. F. RIDGE, Secretary	C. F. LAMBERT, Historian
T. C. WYATT, Vice-President	R. T. LYLES, Treasurer	G. E. BELL, Poet

◀ **1919 class officers included vice-president T. C. Wyatt, professor of pathology at Wake Forest College in 1924-1925.**

1919

◀ **Po-e-try, Phil-os-o-phy! Class poet G. E. Bell takes both to a higher plane in this inspirational rhyme from 1919.**

1918 — Air-mail service begins from Washington, D.C. to New York, N.Y.; price is 24 cents

1919 — Treaty of Versailles assigns blame and punishment to Germany

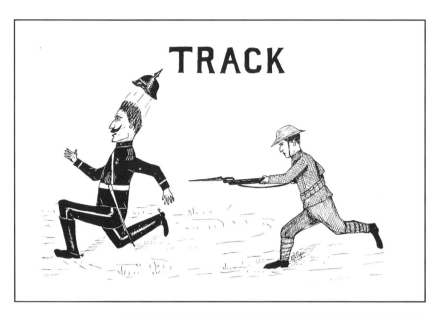

◀ World War I inspired cartoon from the 1919 *Howler*.

1922 aerial view of Wake Forest College. The domed building in the foreground is Wake Forest Baptist Church, and the Alumni Building is just behind it to the left.

▼

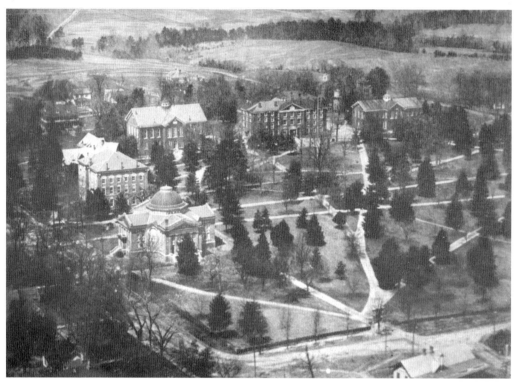

Macabre ▶ humor, also from the 1919 yearbook

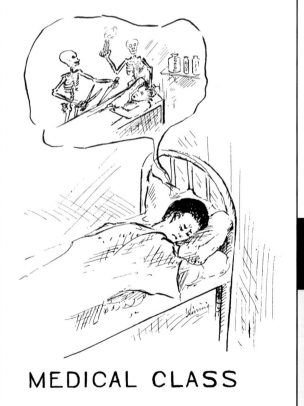

1919

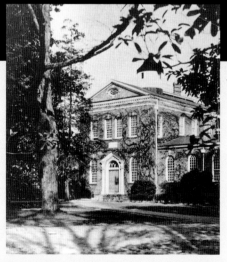

◀ Lea Chemistry Laboratory, on the old campus, in 1921

◀ College humor ca. 1919

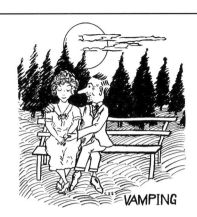

AND NOW—????

Buff Royall (in the moonlight): "Darling, something has been trembling on my lips for over a month."

His Meredith Girl: "Why don't you shave it off?"

* * *

BUT TIME HEALS

Buff: "Darling, will you marry me?"

She: "Yes, Buff, dear, I would love to marry you." (Ten minutes elapse.) "Buff, why don't you say something?"

Buff: "I have said too much already."

VAMPING

Official Rules of the Library

Not more than ten persons shall talk aloud at the same time, and then they must not use stronger words than *shucks, dernit, dog-gone-it, by George, gee, Beelzebub,* and *damfino.*

There must be no smoking of rabbit-tobacco, fig leaves, or corn silks; only tobacco smoke will be tolerated.

Students should not slip out more than three reference books at a time, if the class needs them. Get as many novels as you like. These, however, should be returned your senior year.

Don't register at the desk for any book you want. It will annoy the librarian.

Books in the stack room are for the use of the Faculty only, and students should not display their greenness by asking for any of them.

Chewing gum is feminine. Always chew real tobacco.

Spitting in another's face is positively forbidden. Use the floor for such motley deeds.

Poker shall not be played on the reading tables on Sunday. All bets on the game, when played, shall be confined to $5.00.

No one is allowed in the reading room without hob-nail shoes on. People might not notice your entrance.

No student is allowed to collect and keep all the story magazines for more than a half-day at a time.

Students who go to sleep at a reading table must not be disturbed. It would interfere with their personal liberty.

Magazines are for your use—clip them freely.

A big reward will be paid for the capture of anyone found using a dictionary, encyclopaedia, or other reference book. These books are made to look at.

Fines being imposed upon delinquents for the personal enrichment of the librarian, students are requested to make provision in their last will and testament for the payment of same.

MR. I. M. NUTTY, *Librarian*

Dear Old Wake Forest

Words by G. W. PASCHAL, '92

Dear old Wake Forest,
Thine is a noble name;
Thine is a glorious fame,
    Constant and true.
We give thee of our praise,
Adore thine ancient days,
Sing thee our humble lays,
    Mother so dear!

Dear old Wake Forest,
Mystic thy name to cheer;
Be thou our guardian near,
    Fore'er and aye.
We bow before thy shrine,
Thy brow with bays entwine,
All honor now be thine,
    Mother, today.

◀ Words to Wake Forest's alma mater, penned by 1892 graduate and later historian of the college, George W. Paschal

1922 photo of the College Building, containing classrooms and offices in the central portion and dormitories in the wings ▼

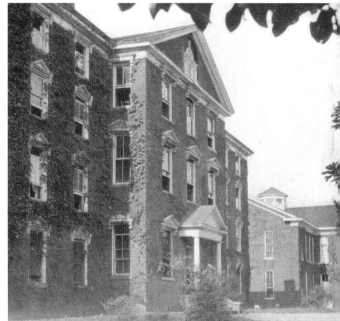

1922

1920 — Women allowed to register to vote in North Carolina

1922 — First documented outbreak of botulism occurs in Glasgow, Scotland

◀ 1919 photograph of Thurman D. Kitchin, dean of Wake Forest College Medical School (1919-1936) and president of Wake Forest College (1930-1950)

1922-1923 — Insulin first administered for diabetes

Sincerely yours
Thurman D. Kitchin

Announcement ▶ of the opening of Wake Forest's 1922 session boasts that its medical graduates are "admitted to advanced standing in the leading medical colleges without examination."

WAKE FOREST COLLEGE

Sixteen Independent Schools of Instruction, Leading to B.A., M.A., and LL.B.

TWO LITERARY SOCIETIES, giving superior training in public speech.

EIGHT College Buildings, including well-equipped Hospital, in charge of professional nurse.

LIBRARY of twenty-five thousand volumes. Reading room contains three hundred dollars' worth of the best periodical literature.

GYMNASIUM with baths; attendance compulsory.

Department of Law

Preparing for the Supreme Court examination and offering four years' course leading to LL.B.

Medical Department

Giving the first two years of the medical course. Students admitted to advanced standing in the leading medical colleges without examination.

Students' Aid Fund

Dr. J. H. Gorrell, Treasurer, makes loans on easy terms.

THE NEW SESSION OPENS
SEPTEMBER 5, 1922

For Entrance Requirements, Expenses, Catalogues, Apply to

E. B. EARNSHAW, SECRETARY
WAKE FOREST, N. C.

North Carolina ▶ Baptist Hospital soon after its completion in 1923, in Winston-Salem

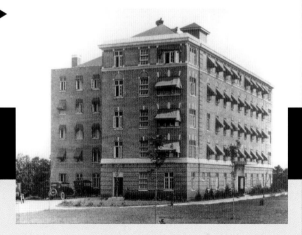

1922

1923 — USSR established

1922 class officers, medical society ▶ officers, and medical student roster. Coy C. Carpenter, future dean of the medical school, was class historian.

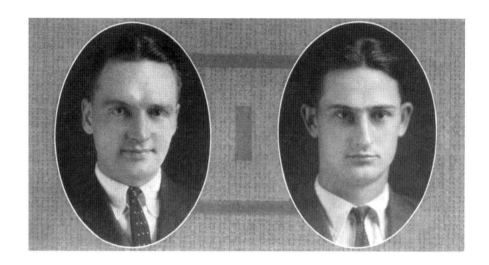

Medical Class
OFFICERS

C. G. POOLE	President
J. F. POWERS	Vice-President
C. T. UPCHURCH	Secretary
E. H. E. TAYLOR	Treasurer
C. C. CARPENTER	Historian

Edgar R. Marshall Medical Society
OFFICERS

C. A. THOMPSON	President
D. BARNES	Vice-President
W. T. WARD	Secretary-Treasurer
W. D. EVANS	Assistant Secretary-Treasurer

ROLL

ANDERS, J. C.	FERACA, J.	POWERS, J. F.
BAILEY, C. W.	GIBSON, M. W.	SHUFORD, H. M.
BARNES, D.	GILMORE, C. M.	STRAUGHAN, J. W.
BARNES, T.	HECKMAN, G. B.	SMITH, W. G.
BAXTER, O. D.	HODGE, A. R.	SIMPSON, H. H.
BEST, D. E.	HOWARD, J. R.	TAYLOR, E. H. E.
CARPENTER, C. C.	JOHNSON, W. A.	THOMPSON, C. A.
CARROLL, F. W.	MACDONALD, F. B.	UPCHURCH, C. T.
CHEVES, W. G.	MEARS, G. A.	WARD, W. T.
DODD, B. R.	MOORE, D. F.	WILLIAMS, W. N.
EVANS, W. D.	POOLE, C. G.	WESTERHOFF, P. D.

The medical school moved from the Alumni Building to the William Amos Johnson Medical Building in 1933. The new building was named for an anatomy instructor who served on the faculty for one year before his death in an automobile accident on Thanksgiving Day in 1927.

▼

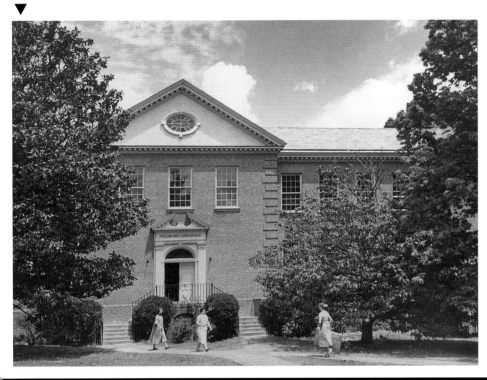

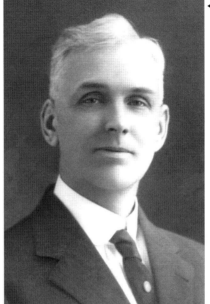

◀ The Reverend George T. Lumpkin, shown in a 1929 photograph, was appointed superintendent of North Carolina Baptist Hospital in April 1922 and held that position until his death in 1934.

Physician makes a house call in this
▼ illustration from the 1928 *Howler*.

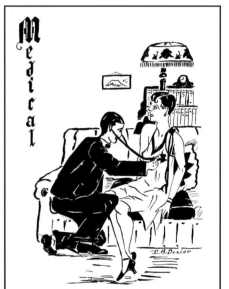

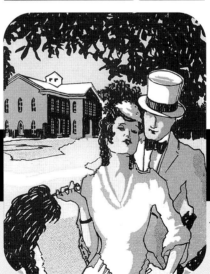

1932

1923 — Nobel Prize awarded to Banting, Best, and McCloud for discovery of insulin

1928 — Penicillin is discovered by Alexander Fleming

◀ Dapper gentleman and elegant lady epitomize campus life at Wake Forest College in this 1928 yearbook illustration.

The 1937-1938 faculty of Wake Forest College School of Medical Sciences meets at the Sir Walter Raleigh Hotel in 1938. Pictured (L to R) are Edward Herring, O. C. Bradbury, Joseph J. Combs, Ivan Procter, Edward S. King, Herbert M. Vann '15, N. Henry McLeod, Robert L. McGee, Loren L. Chastain '44, Hubert Royster, Herbert C. Tidwell, Thurman D. Kitchin, Coy C. Carpenter '22, George C. Mackie '26, William Dewar, and Hubert Haywood.

▼

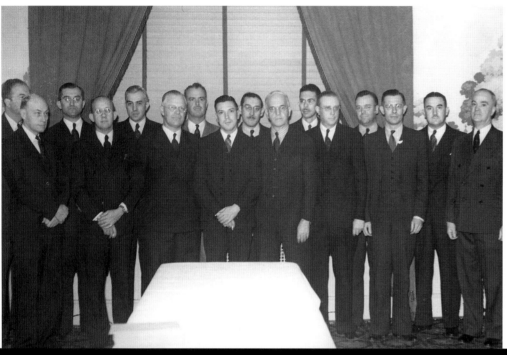

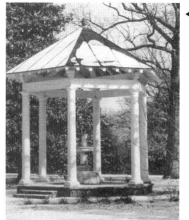

◄ The original Wake Forest campus had its own "Old Well," seen in this 1930s photograph.

Governor Clyde R. Hoey appoints Coy C. Carpenter, dean of the Wake Forest College medical school, to a commission to "study, consider and report upon" a plan to establish a medical school in the state, in this document dated May 28, 1937.

▼

1933

1929-1933 —
Great Depression

1931 — Electron
microscope developed

1937 — National
Cancer Institute
established

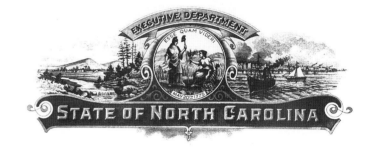

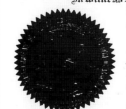

Attending the groundbreaking ceremony for the new medical school in late spring 1940 are (L to R, back row) R. L. Wall, T. W. Blackwell, J. S. Lynch, Smith Hagaman, W. Grady Southern; (front row) W. K. Rand, O. M. Mull, Wayland Cooke, W. K. McGee, E. L. Davis, Sr., C. C. Carpenter.
▼

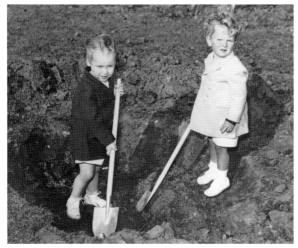

◀ Bowman Gray III (L) and E. Lawrence Davis III at the official groundbreaking ceremony

(L to R) James A. Gray, Sr., Smith Hagaman, Bess Gray Plumly, Governor Melville Broughton, Bowman Gray, Jr., Gordon Gray, and Coy C. Carpenter gather for Bowman Gray School of Medicine dedication ceremony in 1941.
▼

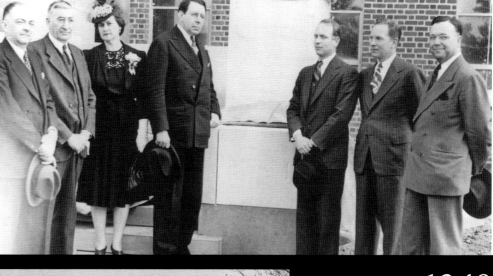

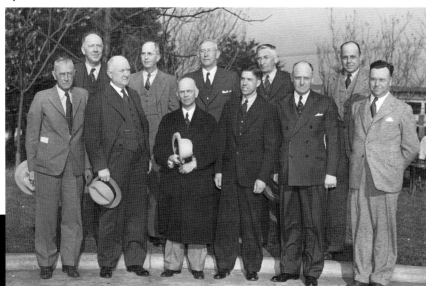

1940

1938 — First total hip replacement completed by Philip Wiles

1938 — First state-sponsored birth-control clinics in the United States opened by N.C. Board of Health

◀ (L to R) James A. Gray, Sr.; Bowman Gray, Jr.; and Gordon Gray at groundbreaking

A native of Winston-Salem, Bowman Gray, Sr., was educated at the University of North Carolina and was first employed by Wachovia National Bank. He joined the sales staff of R. J. Reynolds Tobacco Company, later becoming vice president, then president, and chairman of the Board of Directors. At his death in 1935, his will established the Bowman Gray Fund, which provided the financial basis for moving the Wake Forest medical school to Winston-Salem and expanding to four years. ▶

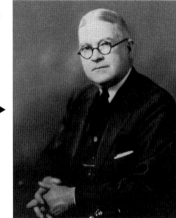

▲ The 1941 medical class officers at the old campus were (L to R) J. W. Rose, Frank Parrott, and Dan Boyette.

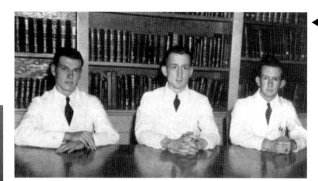

Architect's rendering, dated October 1940, of proposed Bowman Gray School of Medicine ▼

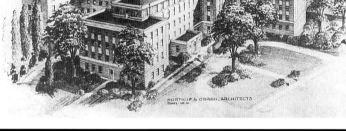

1940

1940 — Germany launches full-scale air war against England

1940 — Hemingway writes For Whom the Bell Tolls

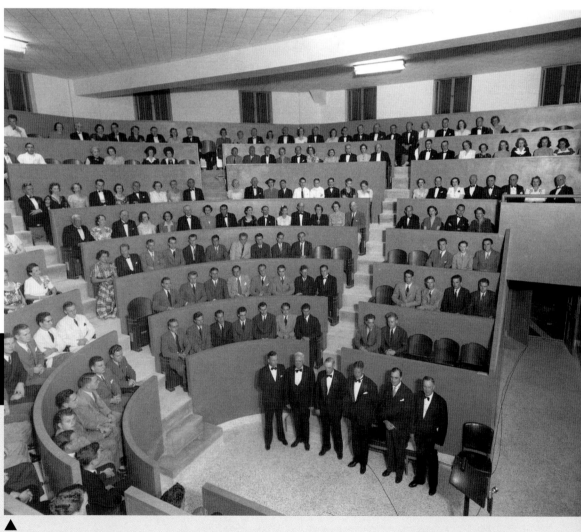

▲
Formal opening ceremony for the Bowman Gray School of Medicine was held September 10, 1941, in the now-infamous amphitheater. Speakers were (standing, L to R) Coy C. Carpenter '22, Fred C. Zapffe, Thurman D. Kitchin, Thomas T. Mackie, Ralph Herring, and unidentified. Fred Zapffe, secretary of the Association of American Medical Colleges, was principal speaker.

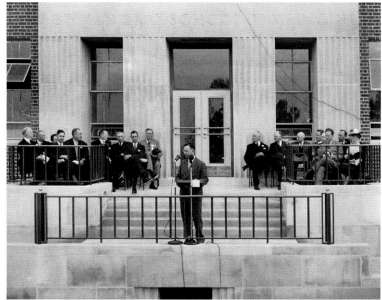

◀ Coy C. Carpenter (center) emcees the cornerstone-laying ceremony at the new medical school on April 16, 1941. Nathan Van Etten, president of the American Medical Association, is the keynote speaker, and the cornerstone is placed by Bess Gray Plumly, sister of the late Bowman Gray, Sr.

Anatomy class meets with Felda Hightower '31 (center) in 1941.
▼

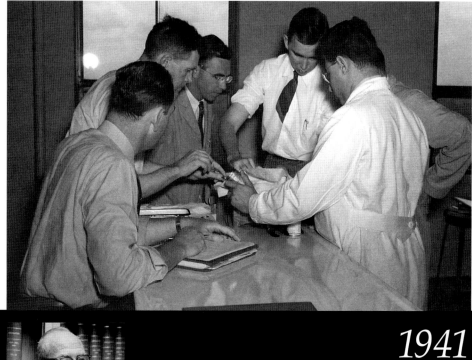

In 1922, Olivia Hall was ▶ appointed first accountant and business manager of North Carolina Baptist Hospital, which would open in 1923.

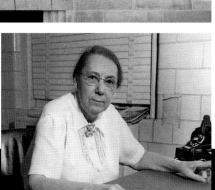

1941

1941 — On December 7, Japan attacks the naval base at Pearl Harbor, Hawaii, effectively drawing the US into World War II

1941-1945 — World War II

◀1941 photograph of Tinsley R. Harrison, Bowman Gray School of Medicine's first professor of medicine

A New Home, a New Name, a New Era - Winston-Salem and the Four-Year School

In the late 1930s the medical program on the old Wake Forest College campus was operating under the name Wake Forest College School of Medical Sciences, partly in compliance with the suggestion of the Council on Medical Education of the American Medical Association and partly because the name accurately reflected the fact that Wake Forest offered preclinical training in the sciences pertinent to the study of medicine but did not offer the four-year M.D. degree. Like other two-year programs, that of Wake Forest College was threatened with closure, ostensibly because of inadequacies in facilities and instruction, but perhaps more realistically for economic reasons related to a perceived oversupply of physicians and the desire to protect the income of doctors already in practice. By 1937 the Wake Forest medical school had produced more than 500 medical graduates, and the dean, Coy C. Carpenter, was determined that the program would remain viable. The best way to ensure its continued existence was to expand to a four-year program conferring the M.D. degree.

It became known that the estate of Bowman Gray, Sr., of Winston-Salem included a sizeable sum that was being offered for the establishment of a medical school in that city — specifically, to entice the University of North Carolina to locate a four-year medical program there. But UNC was not interested in having a medical school anywhere but in Chapel Hill, and Dr. Carpenter recognized an opportunity to acquire the needed funds to expand the Wake Forest program. With the support of The Honorable Odus M. Mull, he was able to secure the Bowman Gray Fund for Wake Forest by agreeing to move the medical school to Winston-Salem. The total bequest amounted to 18,500 shares of R. J. Reynolds Tobacco Company stock with a value between $600,000 and $720,000. The consensus was that $10 million would be needed to fully finance a four-year school, but Carpenter, with characteristic resourcefulness, obtained a loan at 1% interest, using the Gray bequest as collateral, and rapidly made plans for the move to Winston-Salem.

An agreement was reached that North Carolina Baptist Hospital would be the sole teaching hospital for the new medical school; as part of the agreement, its capacity would increase from 88 beds to 300. In April 1940, construction began on the future medical center, to consist of the medical school, renamed Bowman Gray School of Medicine, and the expanded North Carolina Baptist Hospital. The school and the hospital would remain separate institutions but would occupy facilities that were adjacent and communicating. The six-story medical school building was equipped at a cost of approximately $100,000 and was ready (or nearly ready) in September 1941 for students – 42 freshmen and 30 sophomores. The intention was to offer the first two years of medical school in the 1941-1942 term, to add the third year in 1942-1943 and the fourth year in 1943-1944, and to confer the first M.D. degrees in the spring of 1944. But World War II intervened, and an Army Specialized Training Program and a Navy V-12 Unit were established on campus. As a result, the graduation schedule was accelerated, and the Bowman Gray School of Medicine conferred its first M.D. degrees in December 1943. One side benefit of the accelerated program was that income from tuition increased rather dramatically, enabling the school to continue to operate within its narrow margin of solvency.

Despite the institution's unfavorable financial condition, the dean was successful in assembling an outstanding faculty for the new Bowman Gray School of Medicine. Among the notables were Camillo Artom, who came from Italy to the old Wake Forest campus in 1937 and moved with the school to Winston-Salem, turning down offers from prestigious schools over the years out of loyalty to Wake Forest; Howard H. Bradshaw, M.D., prominent surgeon, educator, and researcher; Fred K. Garvey, a Winston-Salem urologist recognized for his leadership qualities; James A. Harrill, M.D., an otolaryngologist who graduated from the old Wake Forest College Medical School and then from the University of Pennsylvania; Tinsley R. Harrison, M.D., who left a position at Vanderbilt University to head Bowman Gray's Department of Medicine and whose presence from 1941 until 1944 enhanced the new school's reputation; Wingate M. Johnson, M.D., professor of clinical medicine, chairman of Wake Forest's Board of Trustees, and director of the faculty practice (the Private Diagnostic Clinic); Frank R. Lock, M.D., who completed a residency at Tulane before coming to Bowman Gray to chair the Department of Obstetrics and Gynecology; and Herbert M. Vann, M.D., who taught anatomy for more than 25 years, first in Wake Forest and then in Winston-Salem. When, in a move both unprecedented and inspired, Carpenter invited any local physician who so desired to become a member of the clinical faculty at Bowman Gray, many accepted the offer, minimizing typical town/gown conflicts and providing an excellent complement of doctors for the medical school. In 1947 Carpenter also hired Manson Meads, M.D., as an instructor in medicine; Meads went on to become professor and chair of preventive medicine and, upon Carpenter's retirement in 1967, vice president for health affairs and dean of the school of medicine.

The curriculum at the medical school had always been strong, but with the move and expansion to four years, the faculty and administration saw an opportunity to test the traditional structure of medical education. Students at Bowman Gray were introduced to applications of basic science principles through specific examples in the care of patients during their first year of medical school. Likewise, during the last two, more clinically oriented years, basic scientists made rounds with students. Furthermore, the traditional strict department divisions were eliminated, and four interdisciplinary sections were established. The first included anatomy, radiology, and pathology; the second encompassed physiology, pharmacology, and biochemistry; the third was made up of internal medicine, preventive medicine, pediatrics, and bacteriology; and the last included all surgery, and surgical specialties. The curricular innovations that continue to distinguish the medical school today can to some extent be traced to this "radical" beginning.

Making ends meet was a constant challenge for Coy Carpenter during his long tenure as dean (1936-1963). Bowman Gray's widow, Nathalie Gray Bernard, turned over Graylyn Estate to the medical school in parcels over a period of several years. The first of these, transferred on September 10, 1941, consisted of farm buildings worth $250,000. This property was intended for use as a research institute, although the institute was never developed. The manor house, included in Mrs. Bernard's 1946 gift, was used as a psychiatric hospital until 1959, when psychiatry joined the other departments at the main campus. Although additional space was very much needed in the mid- to late 1940s, fund raising by the medical school was not a viable option, as there would have been direct competition from a campaign to move the remainder of Wake Forest College to Winston-Salem. Medical school faculty members received no salaries but collected fees from private patients and made "contributions" from this income to support the building programs. However, without significant contributions from the Gray family and the work of the medical school's Board of Visitors (an advisory board made up of prominent Winston-Salem citizens), the continued existence of the school, let alone its expansion, would have been unlikely.

A modest building program completed in 1954 added the South Wing (and approximately 150 beds) to the hospital, and in 1959 the completion of the James A. Gray Building doubled the size of the school. The Medical Center Development Campaign of the 1960s was a much larger undertaking. It included the addition of the Hanes Research Building and Babcock Auditorium, both dedicated in 1970, and the 16-story Reynolds Patient Tower, which was completed in 1973. The medical school had found its stride under the leadership of deans Carpenter and Meads and was poised for dramatic expansion in scale and vision in the 1970s and beyond.

1942 photo of a nurse with an "iron lung," a chilling reminder of the polio epidemic of the 1940s and 1950s
▼

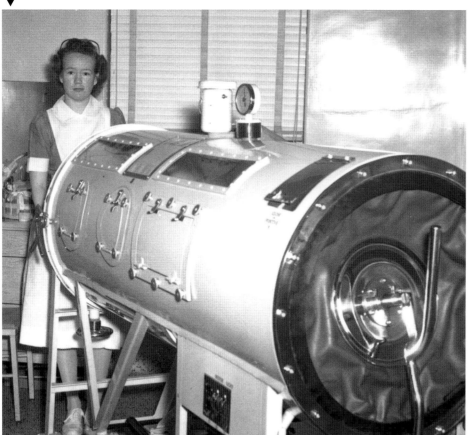

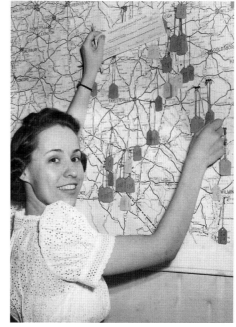

◀ 1942 photo of Nola Reed, first secretary to Coy C. Carpenter and bursar of the Bowman Gray School of Medicine. She married J. Banks Hankins, a member of the first graduating class, the day after commencement in December 1943.

Patient gurneys lined a corridor in the early 1940s.
▼

1941

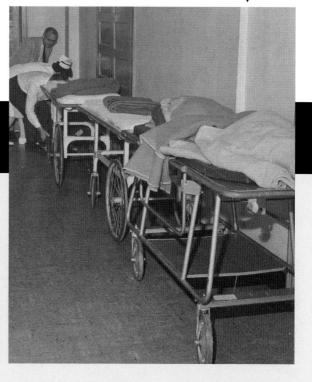

Baptist Hospital got a facelift in ▶ conjunction with the construction of the medical school in 1940-1941. The hospital expanded its capacity from 88 to 300 beds as part of an agreement to become the school's primary teaching hospital.

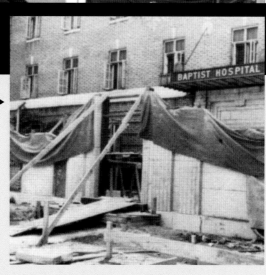

Anatomy class meets with ▶
professor Loren L. Chastain '44
(in dark jacket) in 1941.

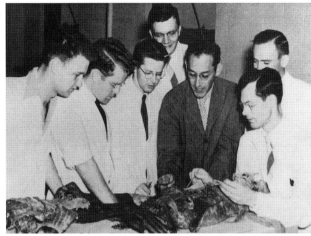

Medical school faculty and residents at Graylyn Estate,
ca. 1942-1944. They are (L to R, front row) Fred K. Garvey,
W. Wyan Washburn '41, Philip B. Hardyman, William L.
Molineux, Felda Hightower '31, Richard C. Foreman,
Guerrant H. Ferguson, Jr. '41; (back row) Ray E. Brown,
Medford C. Bowman, Clifford F. Gryte '43, William A.
Ellis, unidentified, James H. Baxter, J. H. Crampton
▼

Wilbur C. Thomas '37,
well-liked pathology instructor
▼

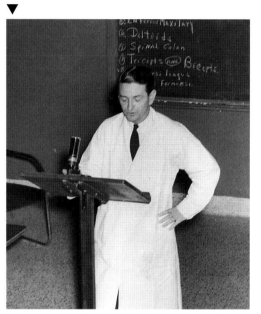

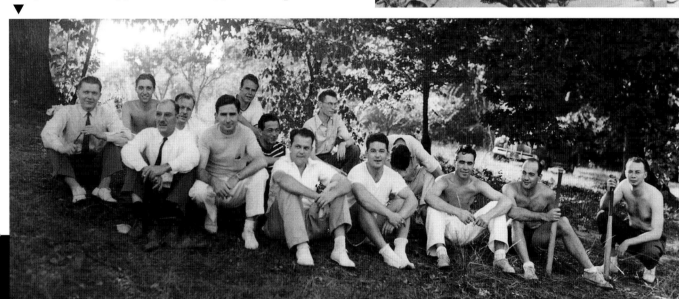

1942

1942 — The first sustained nuclear
reaction is achieved by a group of
American, British, and various expatriate
European scientists

1942 — Nazi policy builds on
"Final Solution" – Jewish
extermination

1942 — Congress of Racial
Equality (CORE) formed by
University of Chicago students,
opposing racial inequality
through nonviolent means

1942 — Napalm
invented by Harvard
chemist Louis Fieser

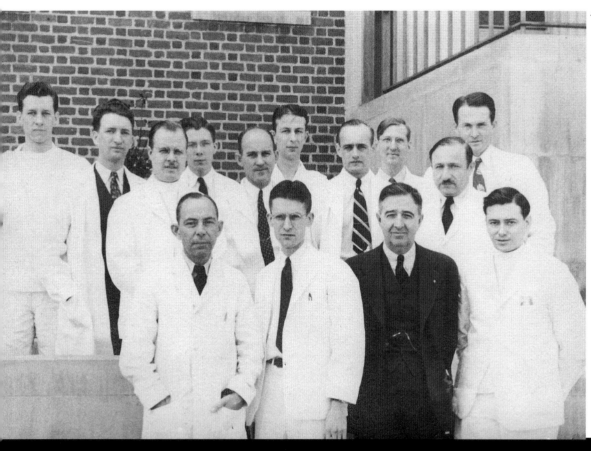

◄ 1942 faculty and residents (L to R, front row) Tinsley R. Harrison, James H. Baxter, Wingate M. Johnson, Charles H. Reid; (second row) unidentified, Clifford F. Gryte '43, Robert L. McMillan, Willis Sensenbach, Arthur Grollman; (back row), Elbert A. MacMillan, J. Roy Hege, Donald F. Bauer, George T. Harrell, John R. Williams, Jr.

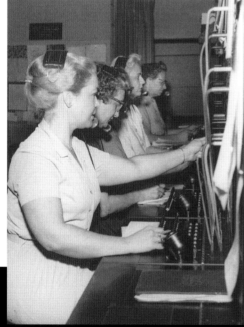

◄ Switchboard operators were indispensable in the 1940s and 1950s.

1942

1942 — A fungus destroys rice crops in India, spreading famine and killing 1.6 million people

1942 — L'Etranger by Camus is published

Ed Rice exhibits ► excellent study habits in 1942.

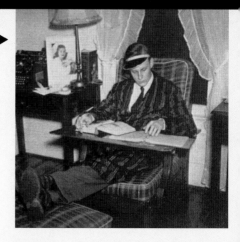

In 1943 Paul Hamrick's Soda Shop in the North Carolina Baptist Hospital was a favorite spot for students and faculty.
▼

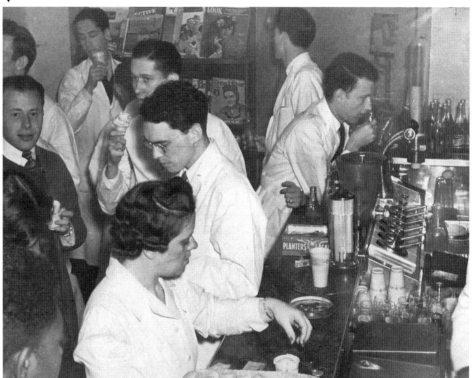

Faculty and administrators enjoying some après swim relaxation at Graylyn, ca. 1942. (L to R) Clyde T. Hardy, Jr., Howard H. Bradshaw, Philip B. Hardyman, C. Nash Herndon.
▼

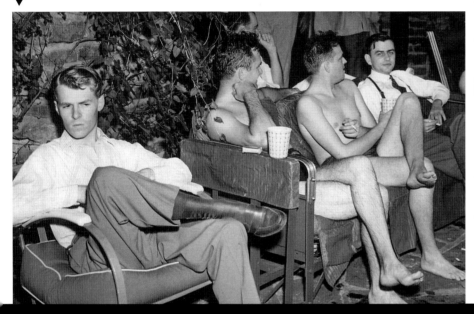

1942

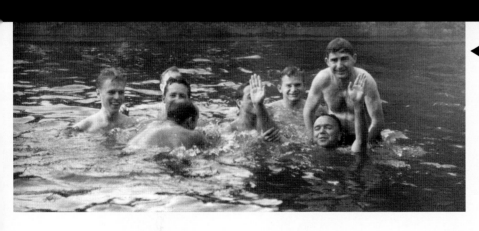

◀ Cooling off in the Graylyn pool, ca. 1942, are (L to R) Clyde T. Hardy, Jr., Richard C. Foreman, Wilbur C. Thomas '37, unidentified, Robert P. Morehead '34, Coy C. Carpenter '22, and W. Wyan Washburn '41.

1942 — US government establishes Manhattan Project, coordinating efforts to build atomic bomb

37

Class officers in 1943 were (L to R, top row) M. Edward Rice, Leslie M. Morris, (bottom row) Joseph M. Hester, David C. Smith.

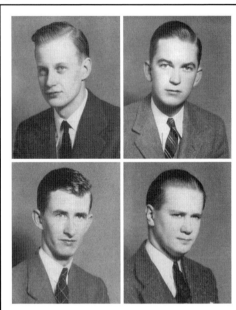

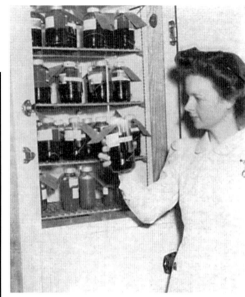

◄ In 1941 the Department of Surgery established the Blood Bank as a community resource. Funds to maintain one unit of blood per hospital bed were provided by the Office of Civil Defense, and medical students provided 100 additional units.

◄ State-of-the-art patient care in 1945

1943

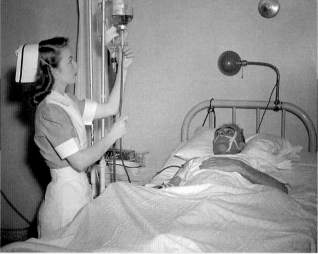

1943 — Doctors begin to use the Pap test to detect cervical cancer

1944 — Board of Trustees at UNC-Chapel Hill approves the establishment of a four-year medical school

1945 plaque acknowledges Bowman Gray School of Medicine's participation in the Navy V-12 program during World War II.

▼

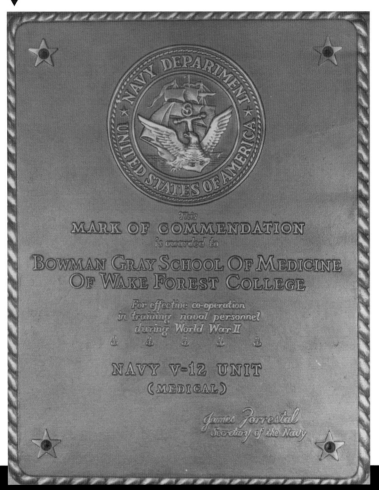

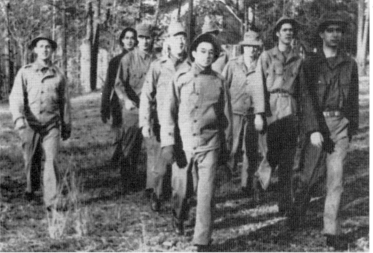

◀ Like the Navy V-12 program, the Army Specialized Training Program, in which the medical school also participated, accelerated the production of medical doctors by graduating a class of physicians every nine months.

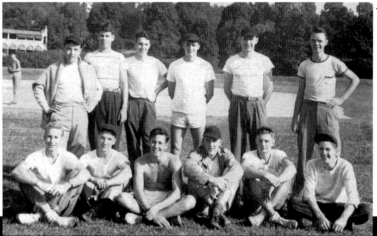

◀ The 1945 Demon Docs baseball champions fielded (L to R, seated) Lester L. Coleman '50, Richard H. Hardin '46, unidentified, Joe C. Padgett, DeWitt Trivette '46, John A. Fowler '46; (standing) Fagg B. Nowlan '46, Norman Boyer, William L. Bingham '46, unidentified, Charles M. Gillikin '46, Lloyd "Gus" Lovegren '46.

1945

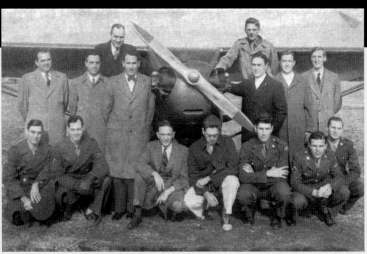

◀ Aerial enthusiasts formed the Flying Club in 1944 with William Woodruff as the leader. The group is shown in 1945 with its airplane, the "Blood Clot" (a.k.a. the "Flying Embolus").

1945 — The war in Europe ends in May with Hitler's defeat, and the war in the Pacific ends in August when Japan signs a treaty

39

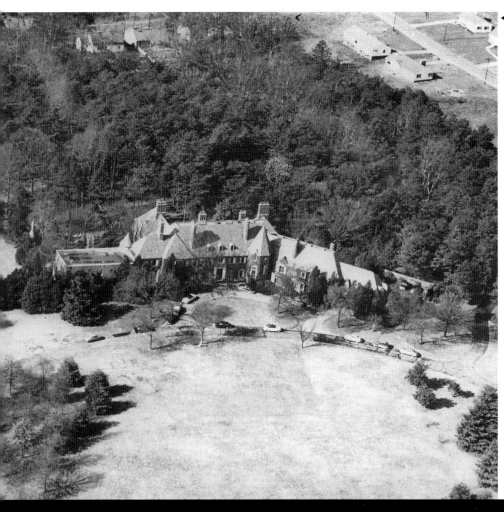

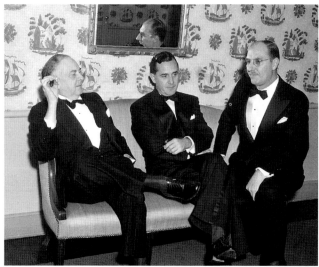

1946 aerial view of Graylyn Estate, donated to the Bowman Gray School of Medicine by Benjamin F. and Nathalie Gray Bernard. The Department of Neuropsychiatry formally opened the property as a rehabilitation center and convalescence hospital on September 19, 1947.

(L to R) James A. Gray, Howard H. Bradshaw, and Fred K. Garvey at Old Town Club in 1946

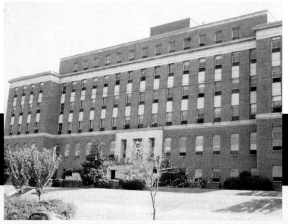

1946

1946 — Board of Trustees of Wake Forest College agrees to move institution from Wake Forest to Winston-Salem

1946 — ENIAC, the first computer, finished by Mauchly and Eckert

Main entrance to the Bowman Gray School of Medicine in the mid-1940s

(L to R) Frank R. Lock, George T. Harrell, Jr., ▶
J. Maxwell Little, Robert P. Morehead '34, and
Robert B. Lawson perusing a publication in 1947

Tote board shows results of 1948 campaign that raised
$1.5 million to move Wake Forest College to Winston-
Salem. Campaign leaders included (L to R) P. Huber
Hanes, James A. Gray, and W. N. Reynolds. The
campaign chairperson was Irving E. Carlyle (far right).
▼

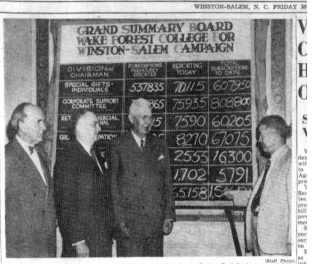

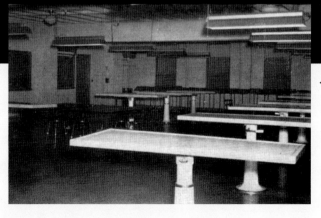

1948

*1946 — Nuremberg
trials condemn 12
Nazis to death*

*1946 — Churchill coins the
term "iron curtain" and
predicts the onset of Cold War
between the USSR and the US*

◀ **Gross anatomy
lab in 1948**

The office of the hospital ▶
administrator, Reid T. Holmes,
exemplified the austerity of the
workplace in 1946. Holmes began
his 25-year Baptist Hospital
career in November 1945.

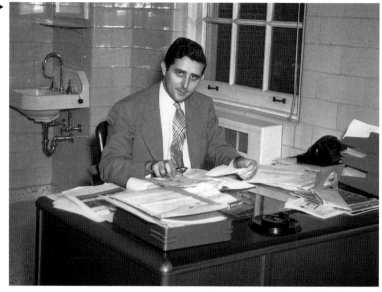

Mary Griffith (right) supervises medical
students Frank L. Fernandez (L) and
Manly Y. Brunt, Jr., both Class of 1948.
▼

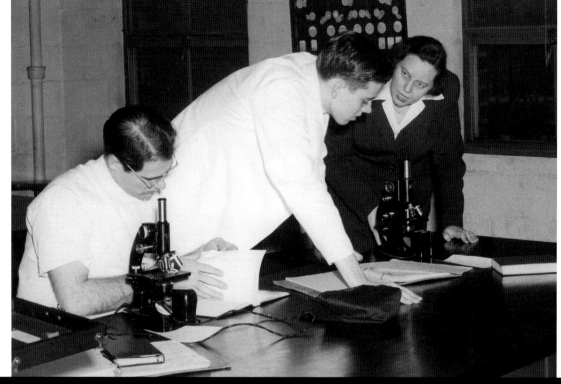

1948

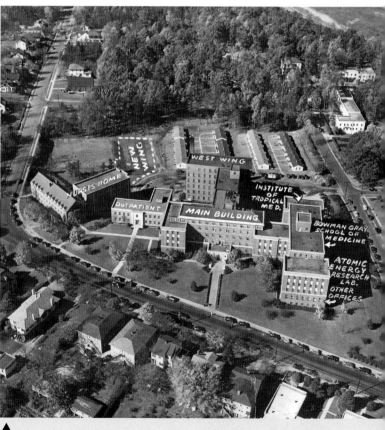

1948 — Mahatma
Gandhi assassinated

1948 — Truman
abolishes racial
segregation in the
military

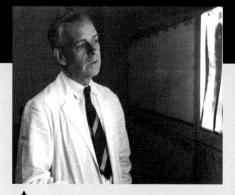

▲
James P. Rousseau, first
chairman of radiology
(1941-1949), in a 1948 photo

▲
Aerial view of the medical center in the late 1940s, with
buildings identified. "Splinter Village," Twin Castles
apartments and "Cloverdale Hill" are visible in the background.

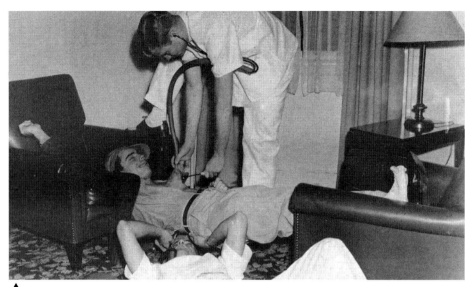

Professor Herbert M. Vann '15 (center) and Phi Rho Sigma members (L to R) John B. Garrett '51, Randolph D. Mills '51, [Vann], Ben R. Boyette '51, and James M. Lancaster '51 lighten up.
▼

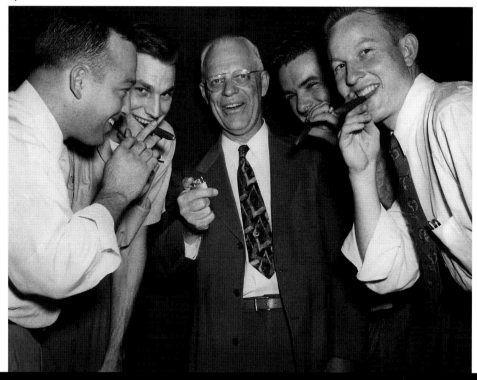

▲
Lemuel T. Moorman (standing) and James V. Sharp perform in the 1948 senior play, along with unidentified thespian in the foreground.

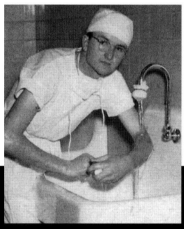

William J. Collier '48, ▶
in scrubs, scrubs.

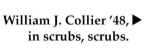

1948

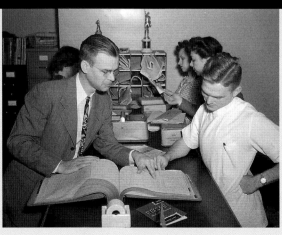

◀ Harry O. Parker (left), medical school controller (1947-1971), goes over the books with John W. Nance '48.

1948 — Activist Margaret Sanger founds "Planned Parenthood" foundation

1948 — Transistor invented; television boom begins to hit: 1 million in 1948, compared to 5,000 in 1945

43

Front row (L to R): Walter S. Lockhart, Jr. '44, Richard Burt (ob/gyn), Donald Whitener, H. Frank Forsyth (orthopedics), Howard H. Bradshaw (surgery), Kenneth Tyner, Harold W. Johnston '43, Fred K. Garvey (urology), unidentified; second row (L to R): Robert Moore (surgery-orthopedics), unidentified, Charles Norfleet (urology), Harold Sluder '45 (ob/gyn), Wayne A. Cline '46, Jesse Caldwell (ob/gyn), Stuart W. Gibbs '44, A. J. Dickerson '48, T. J. McRae '45, Felda Hightower '31 (surgery), Richard T. Myers (surgery); third row (L to R): James A. Harrill '33 (surgery-otorhinolaryngology), William Sprunt (clinical surgery), James Donnelly (ob/gyn), Albert P. Glod '43, unidentified, Thomas B. Daniel '43, Wendell H. Tiller '44, Arthur Valk (surgery), unidentified, Louis D. Shaffner, James E. Shull, Lockert Mason, Edwin Martinat '48, James Rhodes, unidentified

▼

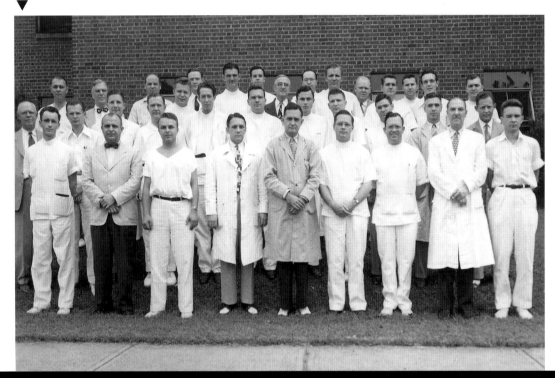

Technician demonstrates expert laboratory technique for early 1950s medical students (L to R) Zeb V. Morgan '54, Spencer P. Thornton '54, and Edward M. Graves '54.

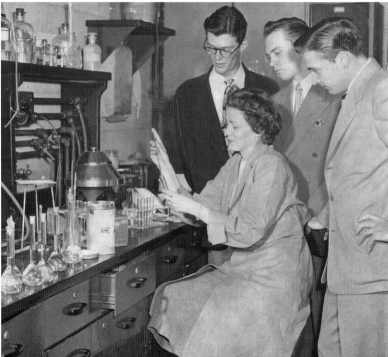

1949

1949 — South Africa institutes racial apartheid

1949 — The North Atlantic Treaty Organization (NATO) is established.

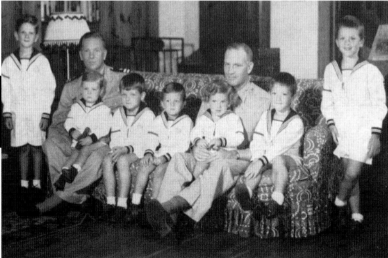

▲

Brothers Bowman Gray, Jr., and Gordon Gray with their children in 1949.

Medical technologists check Blood Bank supplies.
▼

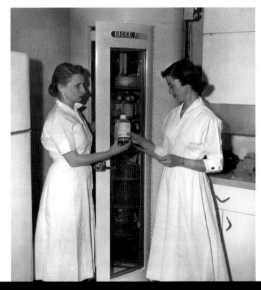

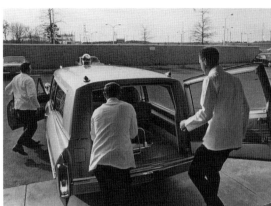

◀ Ready to roll. 1950s ambulance team responded quickly and efficiently to emergencies.

Camillo Artom in 1951. Artom left Italy and joined the faculty on the old campus in 1938. He moved with the school in 1941 and was chairman of biochemistry for 20 years (1941-1961).
▼

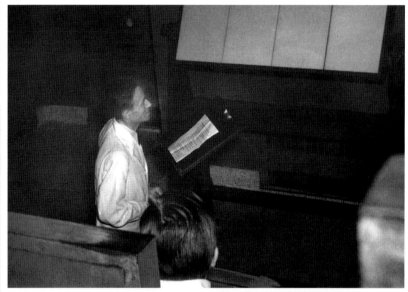

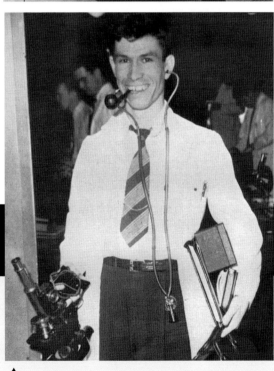

1950

1949 — Dead Sea scrolls are discovered

1950 — Charles Schultz debuts Snoopy and the rest of the Peanuts gang

1950-1953 — Korean War

▲
Marcus M. Gulley '51, well equipped for a typical day, joined the Bowman Gray faculty after postdoctoral training at North Carolina Baptist Hospital and Grady Hospital.

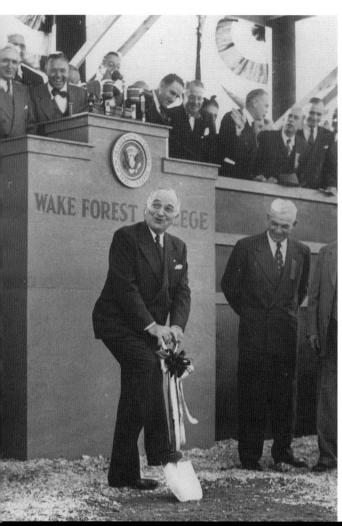

◄ On October 15, 1951, Harry S Truman officially broke ground to prepare for Wake Forest College's move to Winston-Salem. The college moved in 1956.

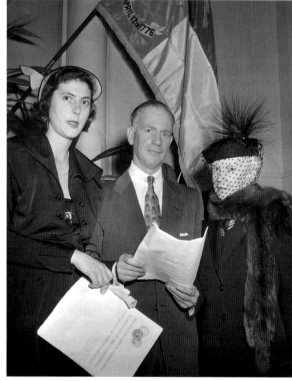

◄ Gordon Gray (center), accompanied by Mrs. Gray (left) and his mother, Nathalie Gray Bernard, was installed as president of the University of North Carolina system on October 9, 1950.

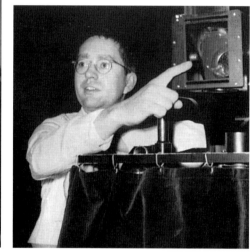

◄

Robert W. Prichard, Department of Pathology, in 1955

1950

1952 — First artificial heart valve implanted

1952 — DNA identified as genetic material

In 1954 the hospital ▶ cafeteria was acknowledged to be the best place in town to eat, and was particularly popular with townspeople on Sundays after church.

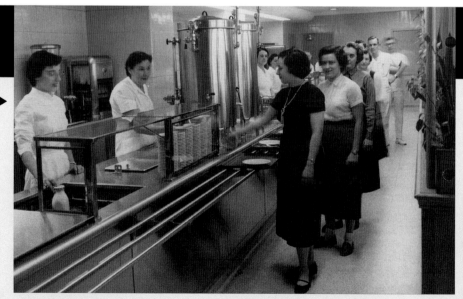

46

1954 aerial view of the medical center complex
▼

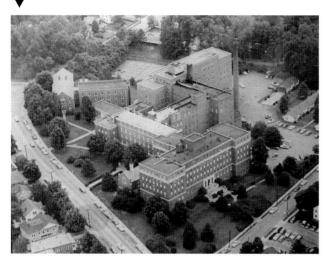

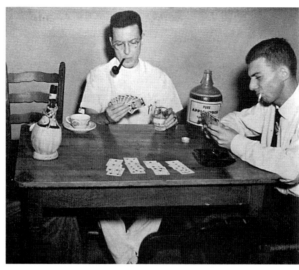

◀ James P. Robinson '54 (L) and fraternity brother demonstrate qualifications for membership in Phi Rho Sigma.

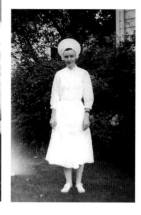

◀ Nurse anesthetist Paulina Whitley Hester, in uniform, 1955

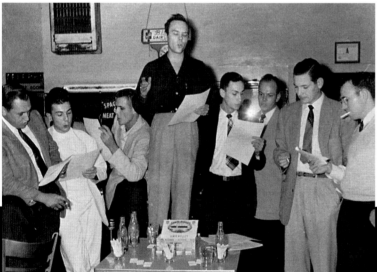

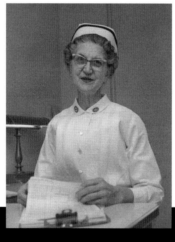

◀ 1954 photograph of Lucia Shirley, director of operating room nurses—graduated from NCBH School of Nursing in 1927 and remained at the hospital for more than 40 years, retiring at age 67

1955

▲

Phi Rho Sigmas entertain potential new recruits at a rush party in 1955.

1953 — Implantable pacemaker developed

1955 — Polio vaccine introduced by Jonas Salk

1955 — Disneyland opens in California; McDonald's opens in Illinois

1955 — First successful open heart surgery performed

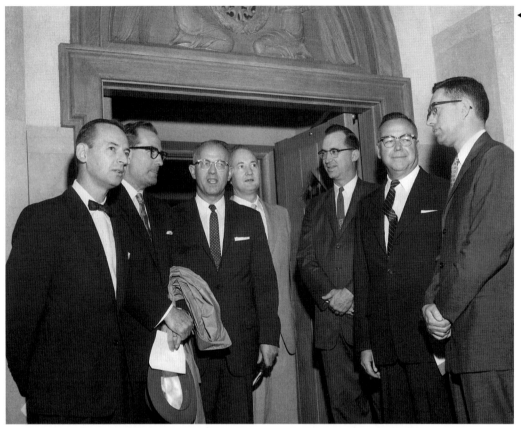

◀ Gathered outside Davis Memorial Chapel in 1956 are (L to R) David Cayer; Rev. Glenn Swaim; J. Roy Clifford, minister and president of the hospital board; William Boyce, urologist; Reuben Graham, hospital vice president for general services; Coy C. Carpenter '22, dean of the medical school, and Robert W. Prichard, Department of Pathology.

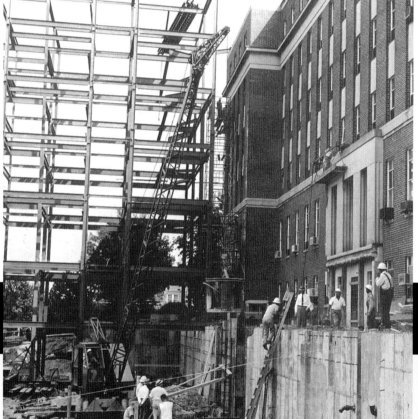

1956

Interior of Davis ▶ Memorial Chapel soon after its completion

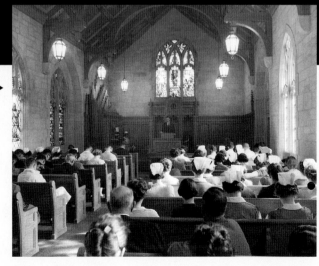

▲
Growing pains: new construction in 1956 obscured the familiar main entrance to the medical school.

The Carpenter family at Christmas, ▶
mid-1950s. (L to R) Kenan and
Harry, Coy and grandchild, Coy, Jr.,
and mother Dorothy

The 1957 Frederick R. Taylor History of Medicine Society is represented
here by (L to R, seated) Louise MacMillan, Earl Parker '57, Nell Benton,
Martin Netsky, Robert Tuttle, Warren Andrew; (standing) William H.
Admirand '60, William J. Linder '58, Leonard A. LaBua '57, Jack N.
Drummond '57, Earl L. Watts '57
▼

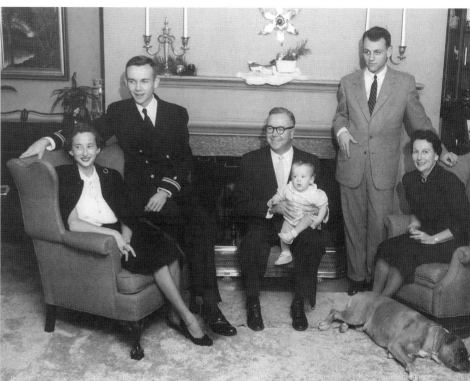

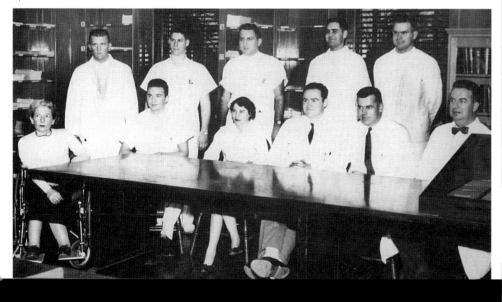

◀ 1957 preparations for
construction of the
Allied Health Building

1957

*1956 — Cardiopulmonary
resuscitation
(CPR) first used*

*1957 — Dr. Seuss
publishes* The
Cat in the Hat, *a classic
in children's literature*

*1957 — Berry Gordy
founds Motown, which
will become a major force
in rock music in the 1960s*

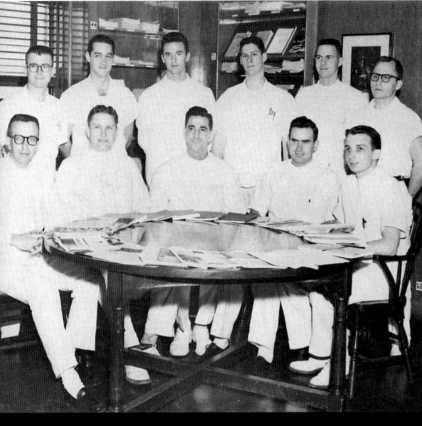

◀ 1957 members of Alpha Omega Alpha (AOA) Honor Medical Society were (seated, L to R) Donald C. Hartzog, Jr. '57, Lathan T. Moose '58, Ralph O. Maercks '57, L. Earl Watts '57, Phillip A. Sellers; (standing) Ed Stevens, Bob Foster, Earl W. Parker '57, William J. Linder '58, Lowell T. York '59, John B. Titmarsh, Jr. '57

Alice Stallings, registrar, who was often the new medical students' first acquaintance on campus.
▼

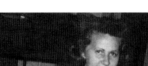

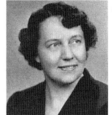

◀ Mary Griffith (obstetrics and gynecology) in 1958. She was one of the first women appointed to the medical school faculty.

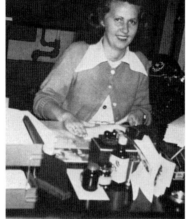

◀ The old Outpatient Department in its heyday, 1959

1957

1957 — Sputnik is launched into the earth's atmosphere, starting the space race between the USSR and the US

Dress rehearsal — taking time from the delivery room to advise class president Jim Jones '59 on the correct way to wear his academic gown are (L to R) Lois Lee '59, Thomas W. Kitchen '59, and E. Terry Davison '59 ▶

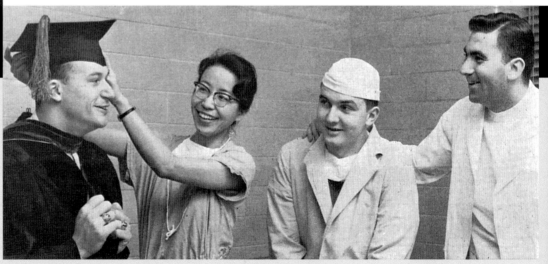

Nurse anesthetists pose with ▶
state-of-the-art equipment
(and uniforms) in 1959.

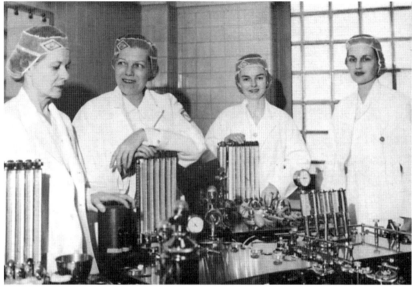

1959 medical ▶
students Thomas
W. Kitchen, Jr. (L),
and James G. Jones
(R) catch 40 winks.

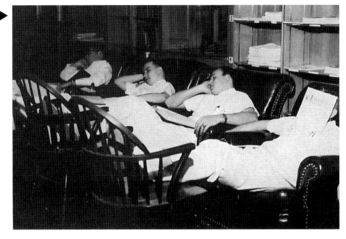

(L to R) Abe Brenner and Morris ▶
Brenner with Edith Gwyer and
Mary Emma Rhodes. The Brenners
were donating a TV to the
pediatrics ward in the late 1950s.

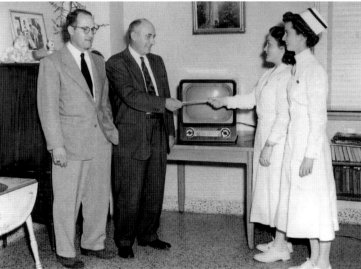

1959

*1959 — In January, Alaska
becomes the 49th US state,
followed by Hawaii, the 50th,
in August*

*1959 — The Guggenheim
Museum, designed by
Frank Lloyd Wright,
opens in New York City
— Wright dies at age 89*

1961 basketball Docs (L to R, front row)
Richard J. Wherry '65, Joe Dudley,
unidentified; (back row) T. Johnson
Ross '64, A. Ritchie Lewis '65, Pete
Rowe, John A. Patterson '65
▼

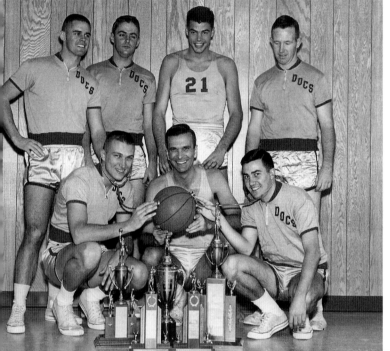

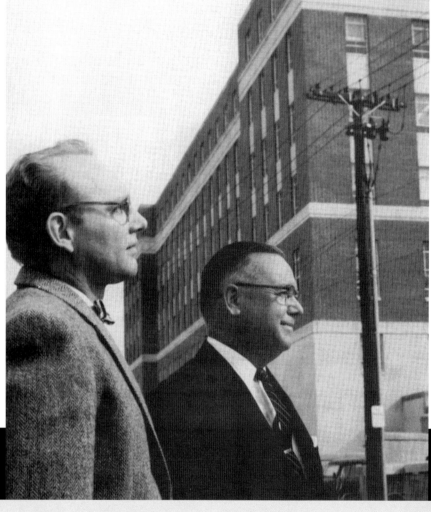

◀ Coy C. Carpenter '22
(R), dean of the
medical school,
surveys the
expanding campus
in 1963 with Manson
Meads, who would
succeed him as dean
that year.

1960

| 1960 — John F. Kennedy is elected president | 1961 — The Soviets launch first manned space flight | 1961 — First lunch counter sit-in demonstration undertaken in Greensboro | 1962 — Use of lasers in medicine made possible with development of "microlaser" by Marcel Bessis |

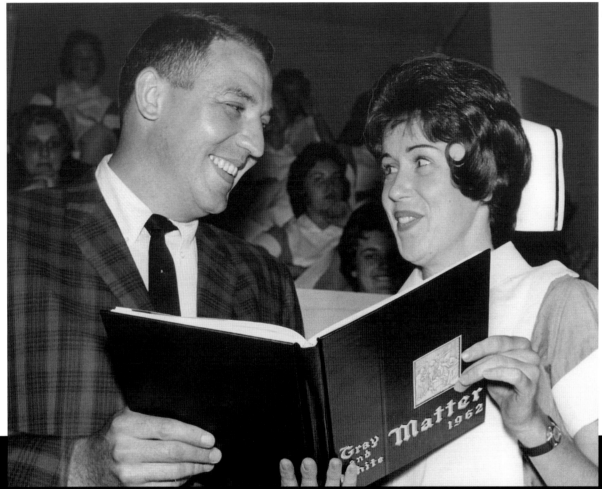

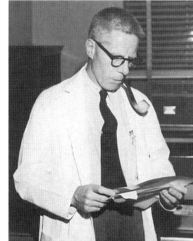

◀ Timothy C. Pennell '60 (general surgery) and friend admire the new yearbook in 1962.

◀ Weston M. Kelsey, chairman of pediatrics (1954-1973), in 1963 photo

1963

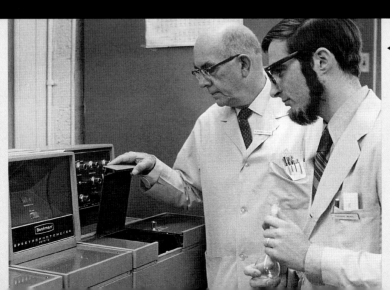

◀ J. Maxwell Little, chairman of pharmacology (1963-1973), and a graduate student in 1963

1963 — On November 22, 1963, President John F. Kennedy is assassinated in Dallas, Texas; his accused assassin, Lee Harvey Oswald, is gunned down two days later

53

Pursuit of knowledge can be a
solitary journey, as Richard J.
Wherry '65 discovered.
▼

◀ Students seeking wisdom
find peace and quiet in
the medical library.

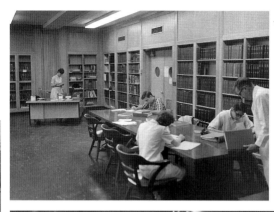

The surgery team epitomized
skill and efficiency during this
1963 procedure.
▼

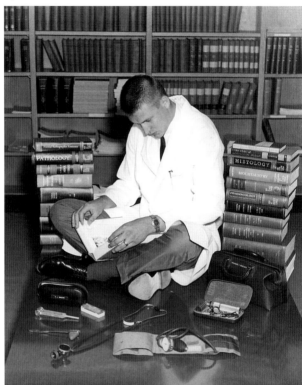

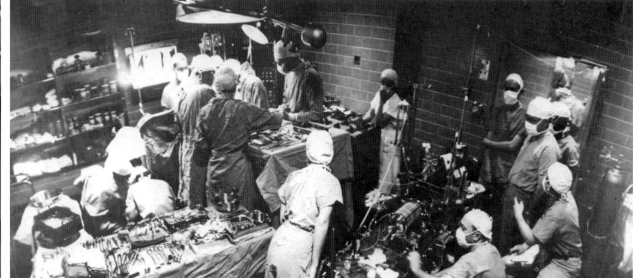

1963

1963 — *Martin Luther King, Jr., delivers his famous
"I have a dream" speech at the foot of the Lincoln
Memorial in Washington, D.C. to celebrate the
centennial of the Emancipation Proclamation*

1963 — *Clean Air
Act passed*

1963 — *An artificial heart is used for the first
time by Dr. Michael Ellis DeBakey in Houston to
sustain blood circulation during surgery*

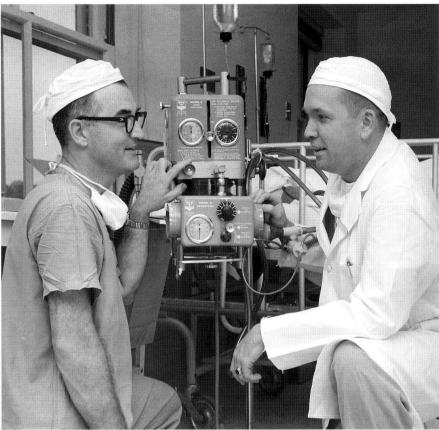

◄ LeRoy Crandell (R), section head of anesthesia, was an expert in respiratory care and initiated this service at North Carolina Baptist Hospital. At left is Charles M. Drummond '52.

David S. Nelson '61 and Felda Hightower '31 compare inhalation techniques.
▼

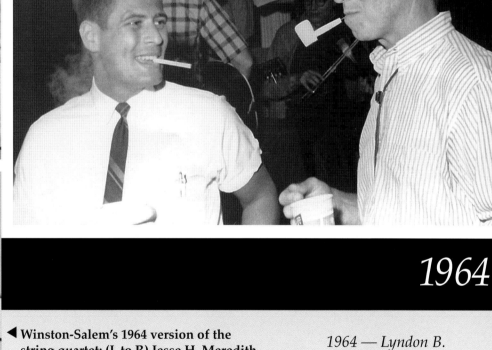

1964

◄ Winston-Salem's 1964 version of the string quartet: (L to R) Jesse H. Meredith, Richard T. Myers, Fred K. Garvey, and Timothy C. Pennell '60.

1964 — Lyndon B. Johnson is elected president

Neurosurgeon Eben Alexander, Jr. (second ▶
from right) with (L to R) J. Edwin Drew '60,
Ernesto de la Torre, Charas Suwanwela,
[Alexander], and Donald C. Roberts '59

1965 photograph of J. Stanton King with
William H. Boyce, section head of urology
▼

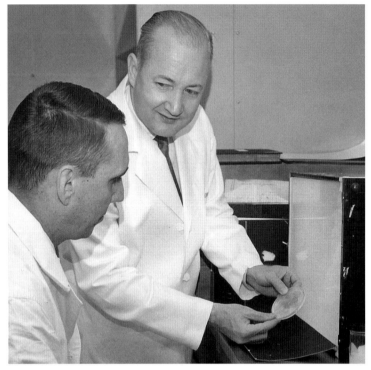

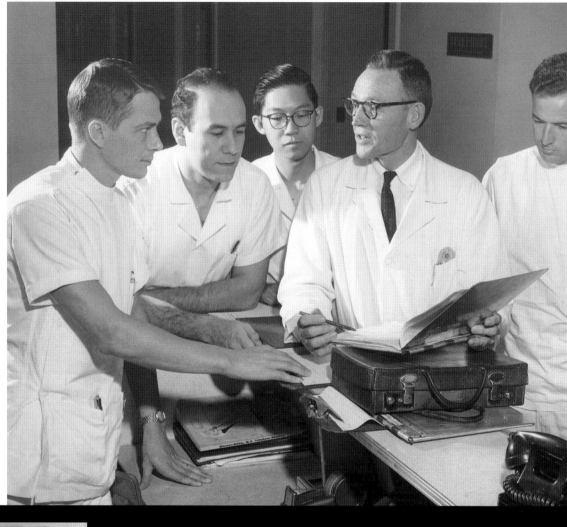

1964

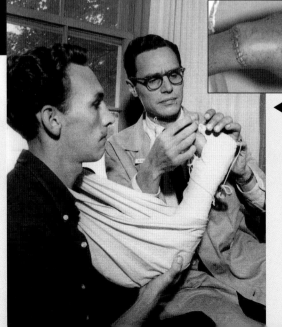

◀ First hand
reimplantation
patient, Robert
Pennell, with his
surgeon, Jesse H.
Meredith. Inset:
close-up of the
hand 14 days after
the procedure

*1964 — After a 75-day
filibuster by Southern
senators, the Civil Rights
Bill passes, calling for an
end to discrimination*

*1965 — Federal Cigarette
Labeling and
Advertising Act passed*

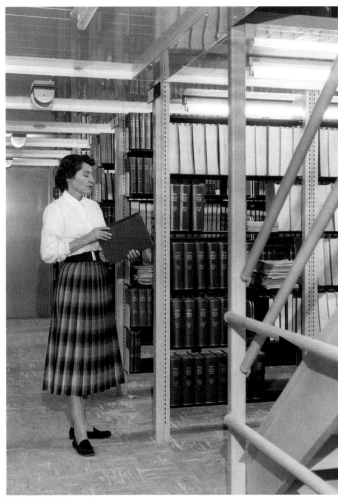

◀ Nell Benton Fuller, librarian at Bowman Gray School of Medicine (1945-1963). Photo from the 1964 yearbook.

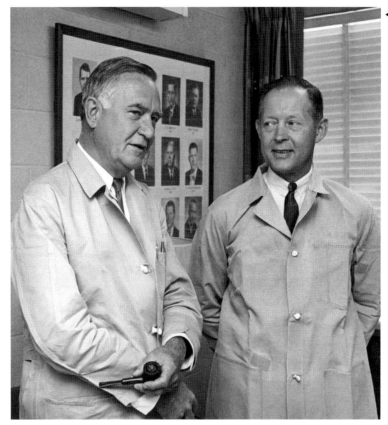

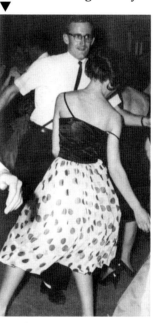

◀ 1965 photo of surgery chairmen Howard H. Bradshaw (1941-1968), left, and his successor, Richard T. Myers (1968-1986)

Twistin' the night away in 1964
▼

1965

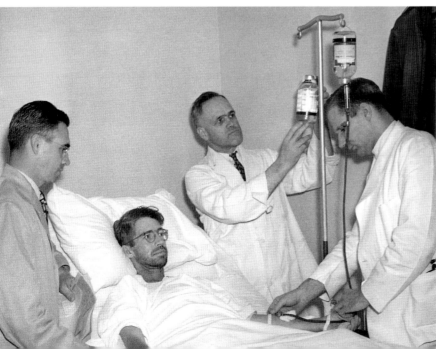

◀ 1965 photo of (L to R) surgeon Felda Hightower '31; unidentified patient; toxicologist William A. Wolff; and surgeon Louis D. Shaffner

1965 — The miniskirt, designed by Mary Quant, becomes popular

57

Julian F. Keith '53, chairman of the Department of Family Medicine (1974-1985) ▶
and president of the Medical Alumni Association (1964-1965), with W. Walton
Kitchin '38, who succeeded Keith as MAA president (1965-1966)

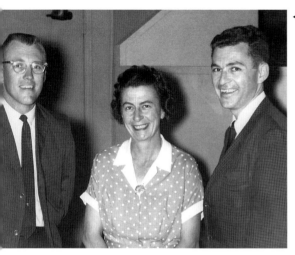

◀ Lucile W. Hutaff (center) with 1962
alums Frank W. Farrell (L) and
Edward V. Hudson. Hutaff served
two years (1953-1955) as interim
chairperson of preventive medicine
while Manson Meads was with the
Public Health Service in Thailand.
She was director of Student Health
Services at the medical school for
21 years and also performed
research in the treatment of
hemophilia.

Richard L. Burt, who chaired the ▶
Department of Obstetrics and
Gynecology (1966-1972), also held a
doctorate in microbiology and
was instrumental in developing
Ph.D. graduate programs in
collaboration with the Reynolda
Campus in the early 1960s.

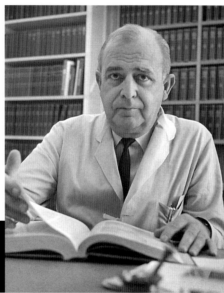

1965

*1965 — Protest of US War is held at
University of Michigan, begins student
anti-war movement*

*1965 — Malcolm X is shot and killed at
the Audubon ballroom in Harlem*

*1965 — Martin Luther King, Jr., leads
famous march to Selma, Alabama*

Joseph Gordon (L), radiologist and ▶
first director of minority affairs at
Bowman Gray, with William
Lybrook and Manson Meads.
Lybrook served on the Board
of Visitors (1961-1981).

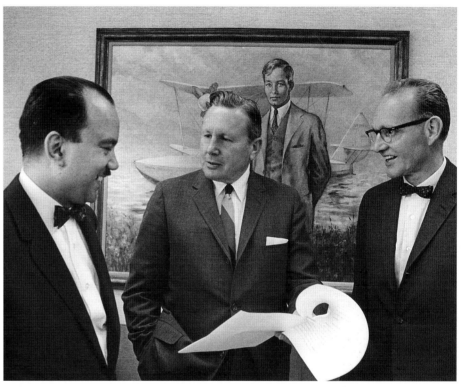

Richard L. Masland (L) with 1944 graduate Walter Lockhart and a nurse
at a 1950s-era EEG machine. Masland, section head of neurology, left the
school in 1957 to become assistant director of the National Institute of
Neurologic Diseases and Blindness.
▼

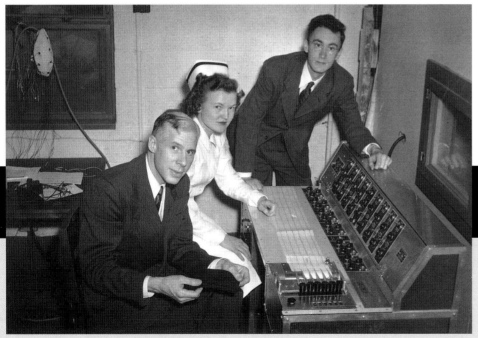

1965

1965 — Ralph Nader publishes
Unsafe at Any Speed, *urging
consumer protection from
unsafe vehicles*

1965 — *The war in
Vietnam escalates, and
American bombing of
North Vietnam begins*

John H. Felts, Jr., (L) of the Department of Medicine, appointed associate dean for admissions in 1978, confers with Colin Stokes (center) and Ernest H. Yount, Jr. Stokes, president and CEO of R.J. Reynolds Tobacco Company, was a member of the hospital's Board of Trustees and of the Medical Center's Board of Visitors. Yount was chair of medicine (1952-1972).
▼

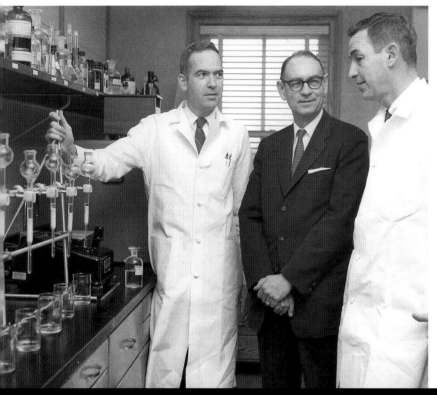

◄ (L to R) Harold D. Green, chair of physiology and pharmacology (1944-1963); Felda Hightower '31, highly regarded faculty surgeon; and Cornelius F. Strittmatter IV, chair of biochemistry (1961-1978)

◄ Orthopedist Frank Forsyth (L) and Anne Reynolds Forsyth, former member of the Board of Visitors, at the 1967 Alumni Reunion

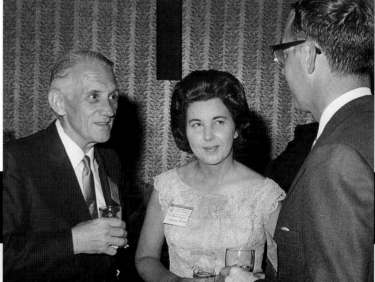

1966

1966 — Black Panthers, a militant civil rights group, forms in US

1966 — France withdraws from NATO, and De Gaulle calls for European union free of US and USSR

◄ Gordon Hanes, general cochairman of the Medical Center Development Campaign, an ambitious and successful fund-raising effort launched October 19, 1963

James A. Harrill '33 (L), a Winston-Salem ear, nose, and throat specialist, who moved his practice to Bowman Gray in July 1942 ▼

Savannah Williams, who retired in December 1965 after 23 years of service to the medical school. The 1966 yearbook summarized his positions as "custodian, chief of custodial services, plumber, carpenter, electrician, embalmer, diener, cremator, errand runner, delivery man, friend, and philosopher." ▼

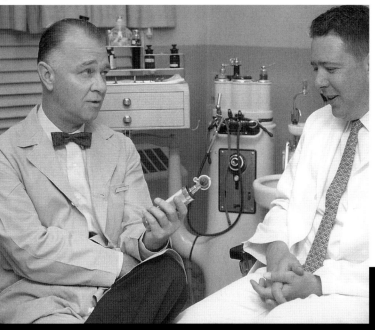

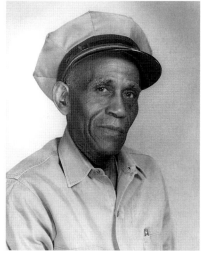

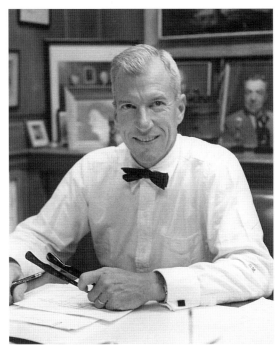

1966

◄ Mandatory bussing – 1968 graduate receives a well-deserved kiss.

1966 — Department of the Interior publishes first endangered species list

1966 — Star Trek begins airing on NBC

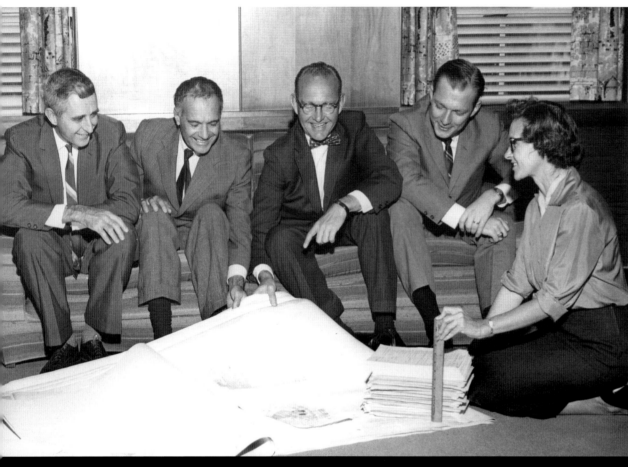

◄ (L to R) Reid T. Holmes, hospital administrator (1945-1970); the architect; Manson Meads, dean and vice president for health affairs; Chris Clark, assistant administrator; and Katherine Davis, assistant to the dean, ensuring that construction plans measure up, ca. 1965-1966

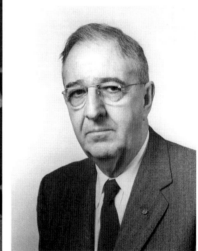

◄

Wingate M. Johnson, first of the Winston-Salem community physicians to have an office at Bowman Gray School of Medicine (in 1942), was a member of the internal medicine faculty, director of the Private Diagnostic Clinic, and editor of the *North Carolina Medical Journal*.

1966

1966 — Supreme Court upholds rights of police suspects in Miranda vs. Arizona, leading to Miranda rights

1966 — Indira Gandhi becomes Prime Minister of India

C. Nash Herndon took over the ▶ genetics program, one of the first in the U.S., in 1943 and became head of the Outpatient Department in 1946. He also served as associate dean for research development.

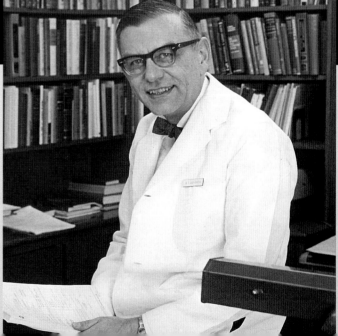

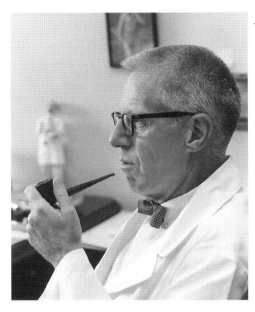

◀ Weston M. Kelsey joined the faculty in pediatrics shortly after World War II and chaired the department for nearly 20 years (1954-1973).

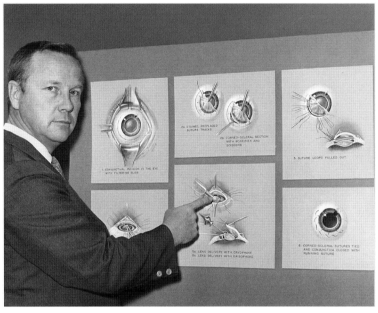

◀ George C. Lynch, professor of medical illustration and chairman of audio-visual resources, who served on the faculty for 37 years. A grant he obtained in the early 1960s enabled him to establish an institution-wide educational television network.

◀ Robert H. Headly, chief of professional services (1977-1982) and section head of cardiology until 1984

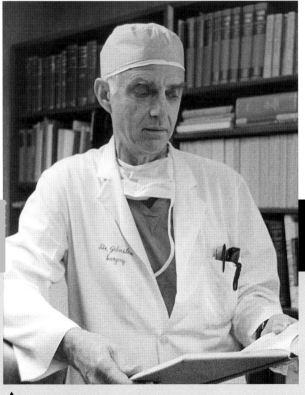

▲
Frank R. Johnston, Department of Surgery, in 1967 studying a medical record in the department library, fifth floor, Gray Building

1967

1967 — Thurgood Marshall becomes first Black justice on the Supreme Court

1967 — 6-Day war ends on June 11 with Israel capturing Jerusalem and Golan Heights, guaranteeing freedom of access to all holy sites to people of all faiths

◀ **Advertisement showing support from business community, 1967**

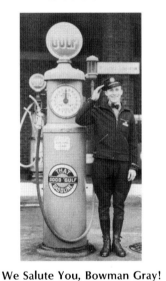

Traditions of Service
Traditions of Excellence

We Salute You, Bowman Gray!
Good Luck, God Bless, Come See Us.
Bob's Gulf Service
Corner of 1st and Hawthorne

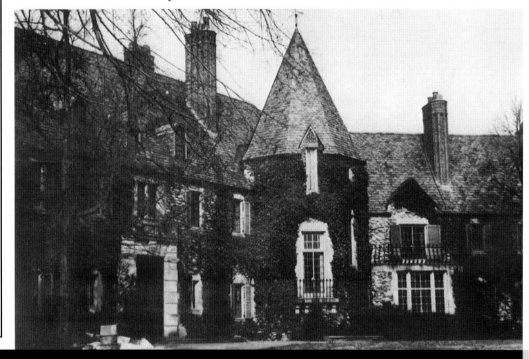

◀ **Entrance to the manor house on Graylyn Estate, a gift to the School of Medicine from Nathalie Gray Bernard, widow of Bowman Gray, Sr. Although plans to develop a research center on the estate did not work out, Graylyn was put to use as a neuropsychiatric hospital 1947-1959 and is now a conference center serving Wake Forest University.**

George Black's family made the bricks used in the construction of the first Baptist Hospital building, Old Main, which was completed in 1923. Here he observes the demolition of the original structure in 1967 to allow expansion and modernization of the medical center.
▼

1967

1967 — Rioting for civil rights increases, killing 77 and injuring 4,000

1967 — First issue of Rolling Stone *published*

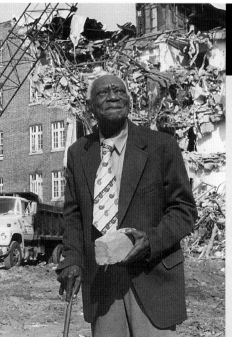

Edwin Martinat '48, director of an endowed program in physical medicine and rehabilitation established by the family of R. Gardner Kellogg in 1962 ▼

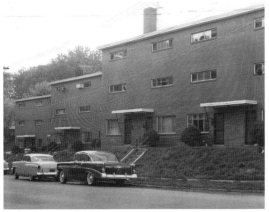

◀ Medical Foundation Apartments at Queen Street and Lockland Avenue, built in 1956 with Foundation funds "to aid the [school and hospital] in the education of physicians"

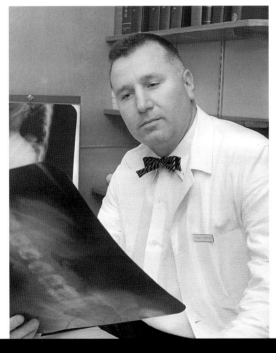

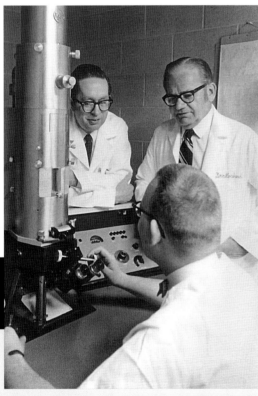

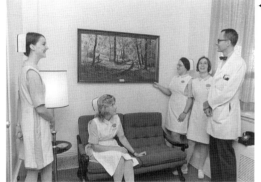

◀ Nurses chat with pediatric oncologist Richard B. Patterson (far right) in the pediatrics counseling room.

◀ Pathology chairmen Robert W. Prichard (L) and Robert P. Morehead '34 (top right). Prichard was chair 1973-1995, succeeding Morehead (1946-1973).

1967

1967 — First heart transplant performed by Christian Barnard

1967 — Martin Luther King, Jr., escalates calls for draft evasion – 150,000 protest outside the Pentagon

(L to R) Reid T. Holmes, Bowman Gray III, and Manson Meads viewing architect's renderings and model for the Medical Center Development Program ▼

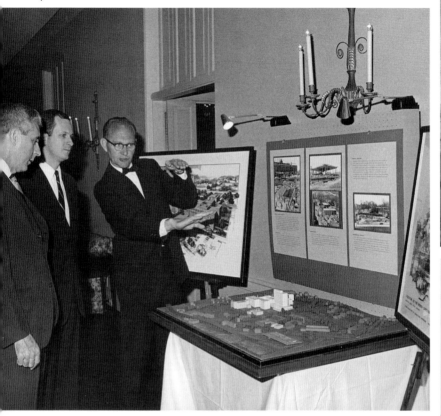

◀ Richard C. Proctor '45, who chaired the Department of Psychiatry (1965-1985)

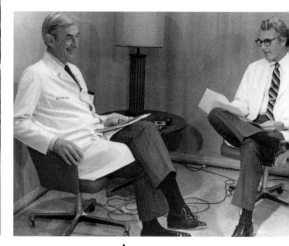

▲ Ernest H. Yount (L), chair of medicine (1952-1972), and Henry L. Valk, a member of the faculty in internal medicine for 42 years, in the medical center's old TV studio on the first floor of Hanes Hall

1968

1968 — Martin Luther King, Jr., is assassinated

1968 — Richard M. Nixon is elected President

William H. Boyce (R), a ▶ Bowman Gray urologist well known for his advanced research on the origin of kidney stones

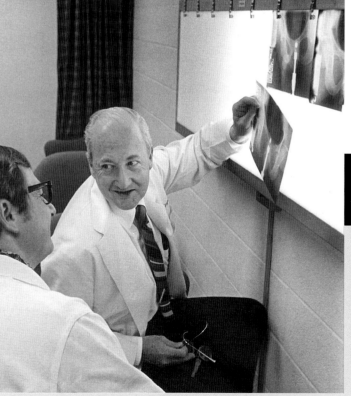

▲ Bust of Henry L. Valk at the entrance to internal medicine department in the Richard Janeway Clinical Sciences Tower

Cornelius F. Strittmatter IV (center), ▶
biochemistry chair (1961-1978), explains
a mathematical concept, ca. 1969.

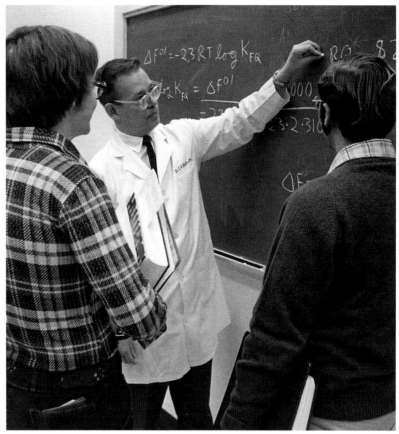

Harold D. Green (L), who
chaired physiology and
pharmacology (1945-1963),
with Carlos Rapela
▼

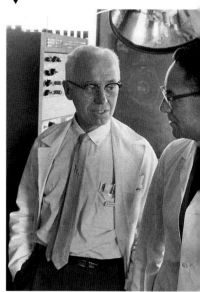

William T. Grimes, Jr. '72 (L), with Robert L. Tuttle,
1964-1969 dean for student affairs and 1955-1963 chair
of microbiology and immunology, in a 1969 photo
▼

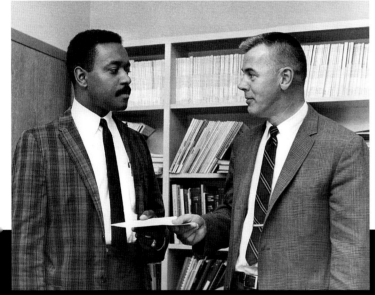

1969

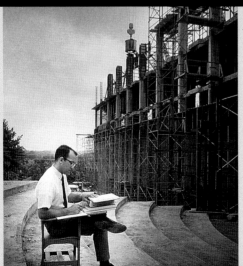

◀ Dedicated student awaits
completion of the Hanes
Research Building, under
construction in this 1969
photograph.

*1969 — Neil Armstrong is
first person to walk on the
surface of the moon*

*1969 — Woodstock music festival
captivates youth for four days*

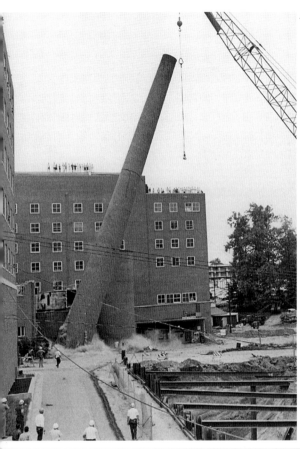

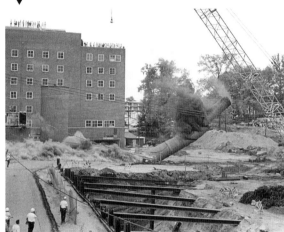

◀ Going . . . going . . . gone! Rooftop spectators got a bird's-eye view in May 1969 while demise of the old smokestack foretold progress.

▼

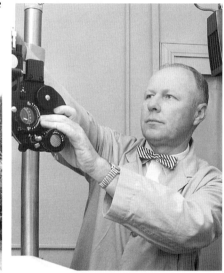

◀ R. Winston Roberts was among the promising young physicians who joined the Bowman Gray faculty in the post-WW II period. He directed the Section of Ophthalmology for a number of years.

1969

The Z. Smith Reynolds ▶ Foundation Board members after a dinner honoring Reynolds Scholars. L to R (seated) are Mrs. Richard J. Reynolds, Richard J. Reynolds, Mrs. William Lybrook, Mrs. Charles Babcock; (standing) Cedric Titler, Charles Babcock, William Lybrook, Stratton Coyner.

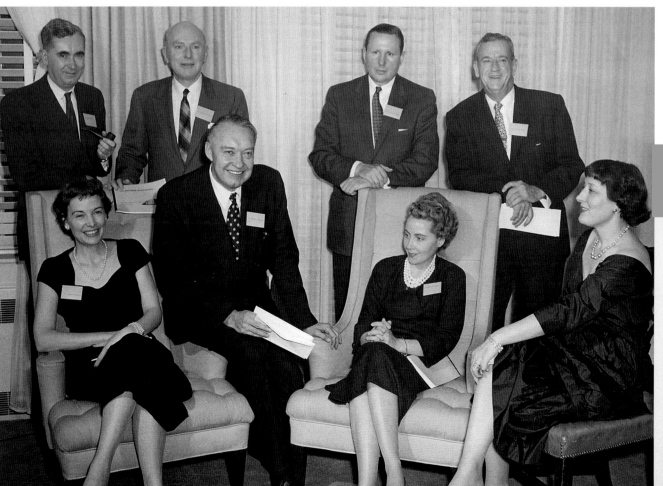

Albert "Chief" Shircliffe, who was head of
surgery research (1964-1988), shown here in 1970
▼

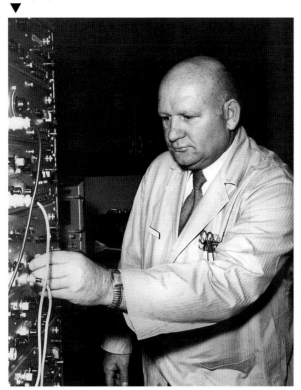

(L to R) Harold W. Tribble, former president of Wake Forest College/University
(1950-1967); Gordon Gray, former president of the UNC system; and Coy C.
Carpenter, former dean of Bowman Gray School of Medicine. Photo ca. 1970.
▼

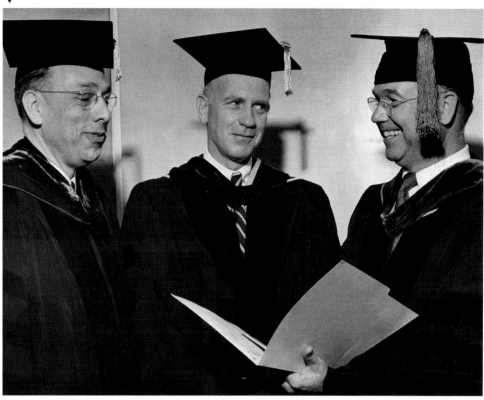

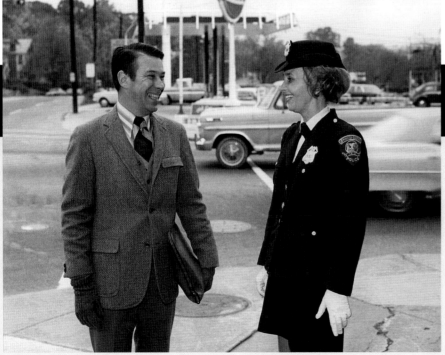

1970

◀ James F. Toole, chair of neurology
(1962-1983), greets police officer
on his customary walk to work.

*1970 — First cardiac
pacemaker implantation*

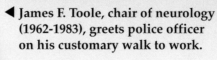

John F. Watlington, Jr., chaired two major fundraising campaigns: the Medical Center Development Program and the Medical Center Challenge. He was a member and later chairman of the Board of Visitors. The Focus Building was renamed Watlington Hall in his honor.

1970 Reynolds Scholars Jerry W. Biddix '74 (L) and Joel B. Miller '74

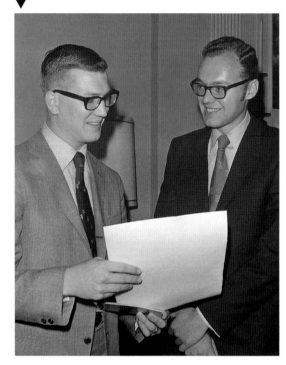

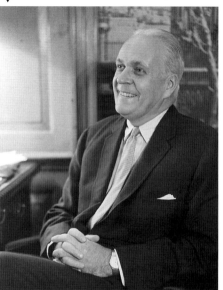

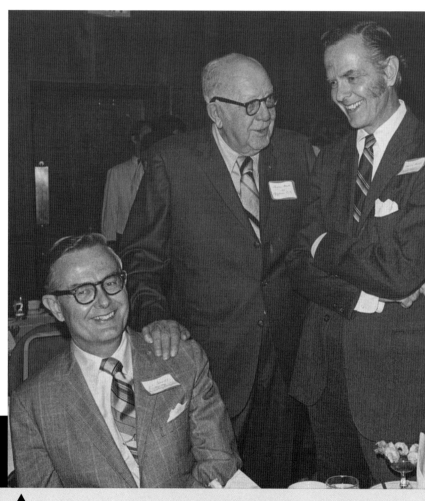

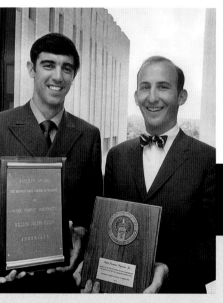

1970

1970 — Occupational Health and Safety Act passed

Julius A. Howell '41 (L) and Charles M. Howell, Jr. (R), with Roscoe L. Wall, Sr., who served as head of anesthesia at NCBH in 1942

Awards Day 1970. William Joe Casey '70 (L), recipient of the Faculty Award, and Sam Pegram '70, recipient of the Achievement Award, have good reason to smile.

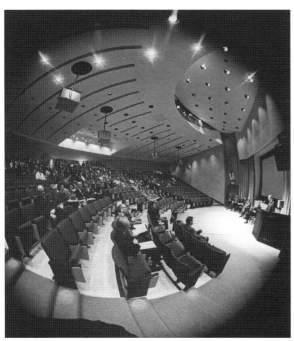

◄ Babcock Auditorium, dedicated in 1969, was part of the Medical Center Development Program, at that time the largest building campaign every undertaken at the Medical Center. The Hanes Building was the other major structure built with these funds.

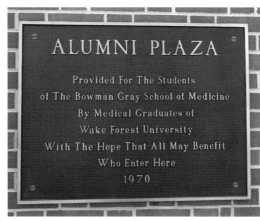

◄ Alumni Plaza dedication plaque, 1970. The Plaza is undergoing extensive redesign and renovation in 2002.

◄ So that's why they call it "rounds"! At left is Anthony G. Gristina, section head of orthopedic surgery.

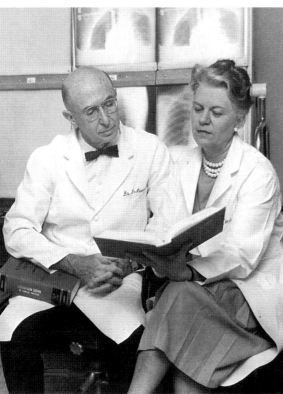

◄ Isadore Meschan (L) and Rachel M. Farrer-Meschan, husband and wife team and prolific collaborating authors. "I." Meschan chaired the Department of Radiology (1955-1977), and Rachel Farrer-Meschan was a member of the clinical faculty in obstetrics and gynecology.

1970

1970 — Student protest at Kent State University in Ohio ends when guardsmen open fire, killing four and injuring eight

The Era of Unlimited Horizons

The Bowman Gray School of Medicine entered the decade of the 1970s with a dual sense of accomplishment and destiny. It had experienced a period of growth in its immediate past, culminating in the dedication of three new buildings. It would be introduced to a new dean in its immediate future: Richard Janeway, a talented neurologist on the faculty who would bring his own vision for the future of the medical school to his tenure beginning in 1971. For the next three decades, like the three that preceded them, the school of medicine would be guided primarily by two deans, Janeway from 1971 until 1994 and otolaryngologist James N. Thompson from 1994 until 2001. Fittingly, Wake Forest University School of Medicine, as it has been known since October 1997, enters its second century with a new dean, William B. Applegate, who had been chair of internal medicine since 1999. The dean's role was ably filled by the former director of the Division of Radiologic Sciences, C. Douglas Maynard, from July 1, 2001, until Applegate began his tenure on April 1, 2002.

Growth of an institution is most easily and obviously assessed by observing its physical appearance. By this measure, the school was in a constant state of growth, as construction crews seemed an ever-present part of the landscape in the '70s, '80s, and '90s. Three buildings dedicated in 1970 – the Hanes Building, Babcock Auditorium, and the Allied Health Building – were followed in 1972-1973 by the phased opening of the hospital's Reynolds Tower, a 16-story inpatient facility that increased the available beds to 655. During the ensuing 30 years, the landscape has become nearly unrecognizable as new buildings have sprung up virtually everywhere on Hawthorne Hill. The expansions of the 1970s and 1980s were made possible by two major capital campaigns: the 1975 Medical Center Challenge Fund, which resulted in construction of the Family Practice Building (now Meads Hall) and the Focus Building (now Watlington Hall) in 1978, and the Equation for Progress Campaign launched in 1985 with the ambitious goal of raising $40 million in a

five-year period. The 1980s saw construction of the 15-floor North Tower, with its associated increase to 806 hospital beds. The Clinical Sciences Building, which consolidated most outpatient functions, was dedicated in 1991. It was renamed the Richard Janeway Clinical Sciences Tower in 1997 to honor the senior vice president for health affairs who oversaw its development. Ardmore Tower with its new emergency room opened in 1996, followed by the J. Paul Sticht Center on Aging and Rehabilitation in 1997. The Medical Center's configuration continues to change, as the new Brenner Children's Hospital, completed in the spring of 2002, reaches skyward, and construction begins on the new outpatient cancer center and an additional parking deck. With available space virtually nonexistent, a number of offices and programs have moved to new facilities away from the main campus.

These changes in the medical center's appearance have been associated with growth in related areas. In the 1975-1976 academic year, the number of entering medical students was increased to 98 per year, and in 1976-1977 the total was increased again, to 108. Non-M.D. and joint degree programs have been added or reinstated, including an M.D./M.B.A. degree and an M.D./M.S. degree. In 1996 a Ph.D. program in medical engineering was approved. The physician assistant program became a master's degree program in 2002. Such changes have necessitated increases in personnel. The full-time faculty now numbers approximately 750. In 1990, general employment at the Medical Center ranked it the second largest among local employers. Since that time, it has assumed the number one position.

Several new academic departments were established: the Department of Community Medicine in 1970, followed by the Department of Family Medicine in 1974 (now combined as the Department of Family and Community Medicine) and the Department of Dentistry in 1977. The Department of Public Health Sciences was established in 1989, with

Cancer Biology following in 1992 and Medical Engineering in 1996. Research centers, often with an interdepartmental focus, began to proliferate by the late 1970s, and Bowman Gray acquired a National Center for Cerebrovascular Research, a Cancer Research Center, and a Comprehensive Hemophilia Center in the 1970s and a National Center for Electron Microscopy in 1987. The following decade saw the addition of a Center for Voice Disorders, as well as a Comprehensive Cancer Center designation from the National Cancer Institute and another as a Vanguard Center for Women's Health Initiatives.

The medical school at Wake Forest has a long history of innovative approaches to medical education. Twice in the past two decades the curriculum has been thoroughly revised. The problem-based Parallel Curriculum was first offered in 1987 as an alternative to traditional methods of teaching medical students. Beginning in the 1998-1999 academic year, Dean James N. Thompson introduced the innovative "Curriculum for 2002," which was implemented incrementally under the name "Prescription for Excellence: A Physician's Pathway to Lifelong Learning." The Class of 2002 was the first to complete the entire curriculum, which has received national praise as a model for medical education reform. In each of its last two accreditation visits from the Liaison Committee on Medical Education of the Association of American Medical Colleges, the medical school has received reports of "no deficiencies." To receive one such evaluation is rare; receiving two in as many visits was unprecedented among U.S. medical schools.

The Medical Center also has a long history of technological innovations. In 1975, it was the first institution in the state to install a computed tomography (CT) scanner for advanced diagnostic imaging. Digital subtraction angiography was first made available at North Carolina Baptist Hospitals, Inc., in 1981, making NCBH one of the first hospitals in the Southeast to offer this technique. In 1983 the Bowman Gray/ Baptist Hospital Medical Center was the first in the state to install a magnetic resonance (MR) imaging unit. And in 1992, the Positron Emission Tomography (PET) Center opened at the Medical Center to provide functional imaging for patient care and research.

The undisputed growth industry at the Medical Center is the combination of research and biotechnology. In 2001 the school surpassed the $100 million mark in extramural funding for the first time in its history. A $67-million research initiative is under way, focusing primarily on aging, cancer, cardiovascular disease, diabetes, genomics, pulmonary diseases, and integrative medicine. We have reached an agreement with Virginia Polytechnic and State University to establish a joint school of bioengineering. Thomas K. Hearn, Jr., president of Wake Forest University, and Richard H. Dean, president and CEO of the newly formed corporation Wake Forest University Health Sciences, have announced a major expansion of the downtown campus, to be developed as a research and bioengineering complex.

In *The Miracle on Hawthorne Hill*, his 1987 history of the Wake Forest University medical school, Manson Meads related a story told by Felda Hightower, first a part-time anatomy instructor and later a prominent member of the surgery faculty. When the intention to move the school from Wake Forest to Winston-Salem was announced in 1939, Hightower asked Dean Coy C. Carpenter how much money was really available for Wake Forest to develop a four-year medical school. Carpenter's reply? "Unlimited." In 2002, as the school begins its second century with a new dean, a new corporation, and new directions in biotechnology and research, how expansive is the horizon? Unlimited!

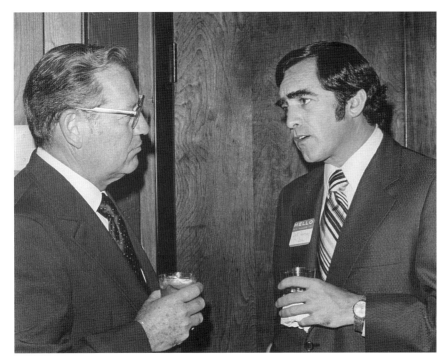

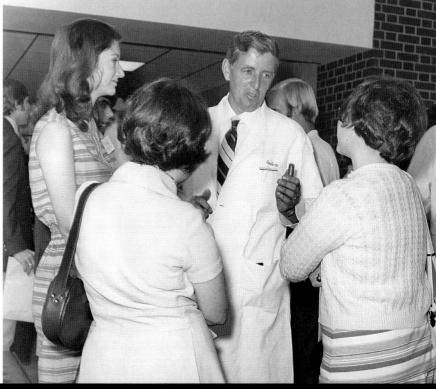

Walter J. Bo, legendary professor of anatomy, greeting students at 1971 orientation. He has taught at Wake Forest since 1960. ▼

Claude A. McNeill, Jr. '43, and Richard Janeway near the beginning of his tenure as dean

Aerial view of the growing medical center complex in 1971 ▶

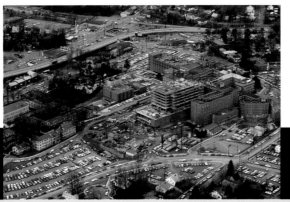

1971

1971 — 26th Amendment lowers voting age from 21 to 18

1971 — Supreme Court upholds an order to bus children in order to enforce school integration

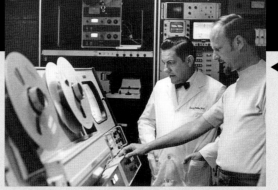

◀ Emery C. Miller (L), preparing an audiovisual presentation. Miller, an endocrinologist, was associate dean for continuing education and later director of Northwest Area Health Education Center. A well-attended annual seminar at Myrtle Beach is named in his honor.

George W. Paschal, Jr., 1929 graduate ▶
of Wake Forest College, and George
W. Paschal III, 1973 graduate of
Bowman Gray School of Medicine

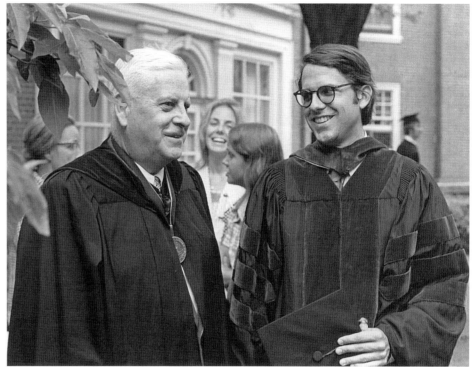

Courtland H. Davis, ▶
neurosurgeon and chief
of professional services
(1981-1986)

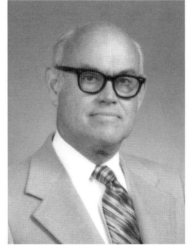

Robert Gibson (far right), faculty
member in anesthesia-critical care, on
rounds with medical students in the
Intensive Care Unit in mid-1970s
▼

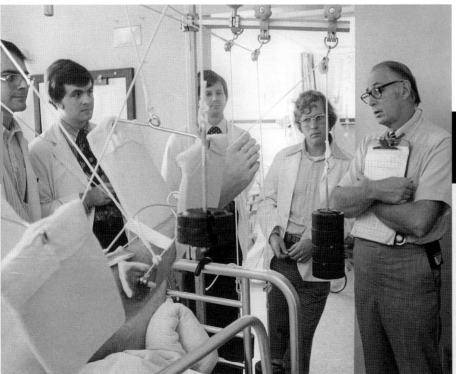

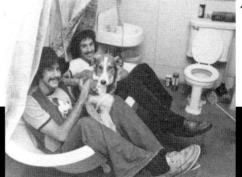

◀ First-year student Jon S.
Abramson '76 (R) and friends
rehearse lifestyles of the rich
and famous.

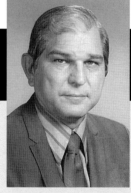

1972

Warren H. Kennedy joined Bowman ▶
Gray School of Medicine in 1971 as
associate dean of administration and
director of resource management.

1974 photo of Congressman Steve Neal (L) with
Julian F. Keith '53, first chair of the Department
of Family and Community Medicine (1974-1985)
▼

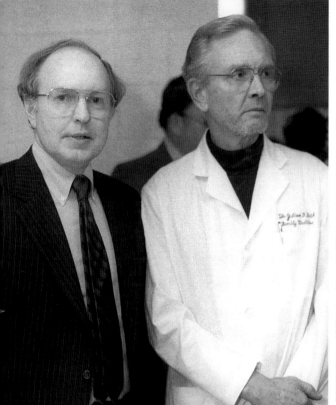

A. Sherrill Hudspeth '53, ▶
cardiothoracic surgeon,
from the 1975 yearbook

Aerial view of the
Medical Center in 1974
▼

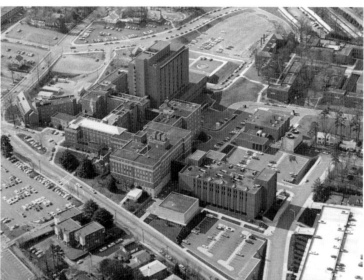

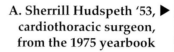

1973

1955-1977 Radiology chair ▶
Isadore Meschan (L) and
radiology professor James F.
Martin show American College
of Radiology syllabus on
which they collaborated.

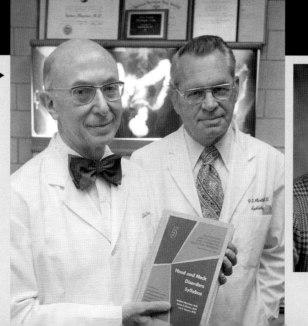

▲
Judy (L) and George W. Plonk, from the
1973 yearbook

◀ Thomas H. Irving, 1969-1982 chair of the
Department of Anesthesia, which began
as a section of the surgery department
and became an independent department
on February 1, 1969. Irving also served as
chief of professional services for the
hospital (1973-1977).

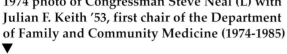

Entrance to North ▶
Carolina Baptist
Hospital as it
appeared in 1975

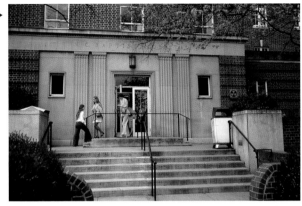

C. Douglas Maynard '59 (R), assistant dean of admissions and associate dean for student affairs before becoming chair of the radiology department in 1977, congratulates Reynolds Scholars Roger Lee Roark (L) and Rosalyn R. Isaacs, both 1975 graduates.
▼

Alanson Hinman, member of the ▶
pediatrics faculty and director of
Amos Cottage, at the 1975
dedication ceremony

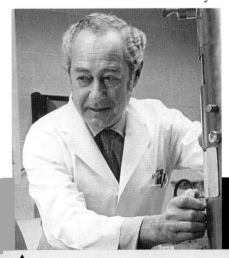

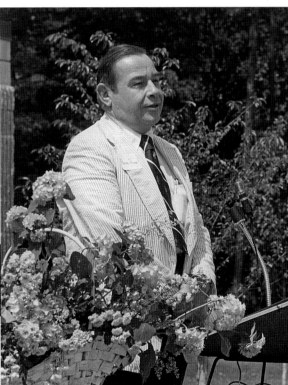

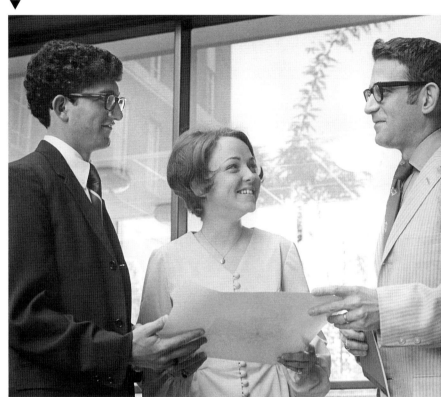

▲
Norman M. Sulkin was
chair of the Department of
Anatomy from 1958 until
his death in November 1975.
A nationally prominent
neuroanatomist, he
developed the medical
center's first Ph.D. program.

Vera Mace receives a corsage ▶
from admirer David Mace.
The Maces, both physicians,
were faculty members in the
Department of Medical Social
Science and Marital Health.

1975

*1974 — Richard
Nixon resigns
after Watergate
scandal; Gerald
Ford becomes
President*

Eugene H. Paschold '78 (L) with Harold O. Goodman, holding Teaching Excellence Award in 1978. Goodman was a faculty member in pediatrics for 33 years, including eight as associate dean for biomedical graduate studies. A medical geneticist, he was an expert on Down's syndrome.
▼

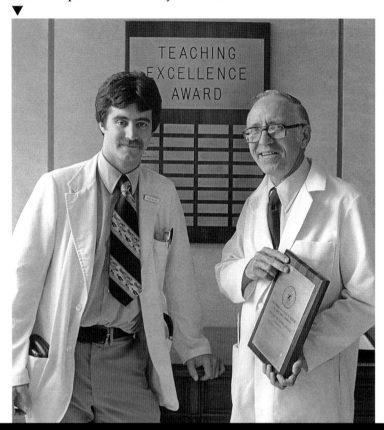

J. Ralph Scales (L), president of Wake Forest University (1967-1983), and Manson Meads, vice president for health affairs (1967-1983) and dean of the medical school (1963-1971). Under their leadership, the university and the medical school developed a mutually supportive relationship.

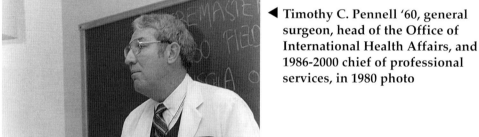

Timothy C. Pennell '60, general surgeon, head of the Office of International Health Affairs, and 1986-2000 chief of professional services, in 1980 photo

1976

1977 — Rock pioneer Elvis Presley dies in Memphis

1978 — First birth of a "test tube" baby

1979 — CT scanner developed by G. Hounsfield and Cormack

Medical Center administration in 1980 (L to R): ▶
Richard Janeway, dean of the medical school (1971-1994); Manson Meads, vice president for health affairs (1967-1983) and director of the Medical Center (1974-1983); and John E. Lynch, hospital CEO (1972-1988) and president (1974-1988)

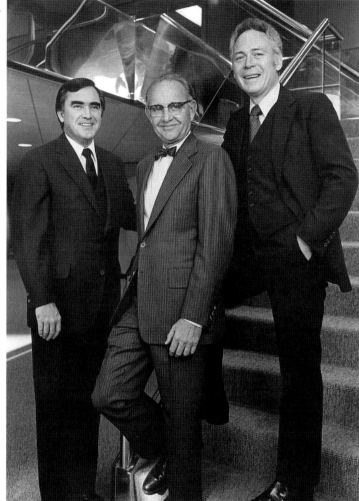

1975 photo of ▶
Elias G. Theros, radiologist and Renaissance man. A multitalented and renowned teacher, Theros was the first I. Meschan Distinguished Professor of Radiology.

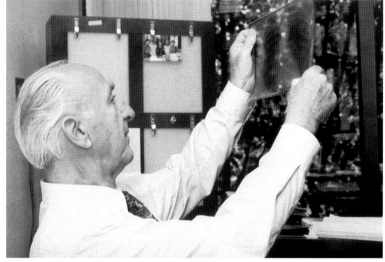

1980

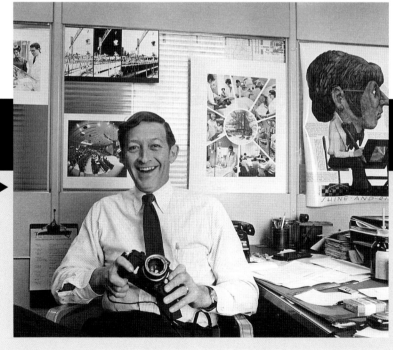

Bill Glance, who ▶
joined the Office of Information and Publications in 1962 and headed that office until the mid-1990s

1980 — Voyager I, a NASA probe, explores Saturn

1980 — Ronald Reagan is elected President

Gary G. Poehling, chair of ▶
orthopaedic surgery since 1989,
during 1980 visit to China

W. Keith O'Steen (L), chair of neurobiology and anatomy for 16 years
(1977-1994). O'Steen was well known for his studies of retinal deterioration.
In this 1980 photo he is seen with graduate students Thane Duncan and
Clara Miller preparing to inject mice with hormones.
▼

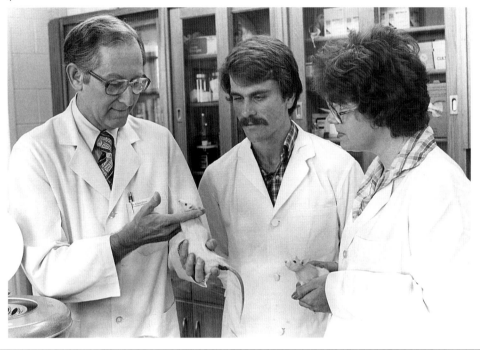

1980

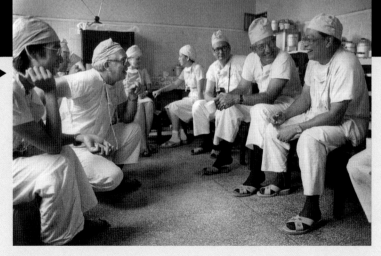

After observing ▶
surgeon David
Fong (far right)
perform a heart
valve replacement,
American
physicians sit
down for tea and
discussion.

*1980 — Lech Walesa leads a
strike by Polish shipyard workers
and forms an independent labor
union, outside of Soviet influence*

*1980 — In the state
of Washington,
Mt. St. Helens erupts*

George Herbert Walker Bush, then Vice President, greets Manson Meads (R), dean of the medical school (1963-1971) during the Medical Center's 40th anniversary celebration in 1981. In the background are (L to R) Kathy Janeway, John Lynch, president of North Carolina Baptist Hospital (1970-1988), and Beth Lynch.

▼

▶ This computed tomography (CT) scanner was manufactured by EMI, a company backed financially by the Beatles. The first CT scanner in the state was installed at the Medical Center in 1975.

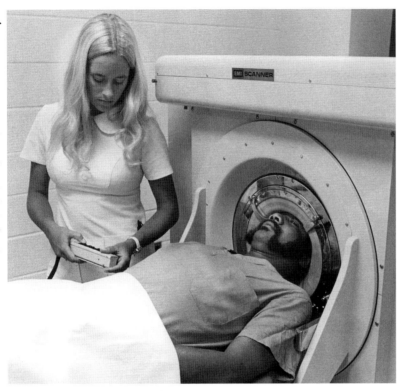

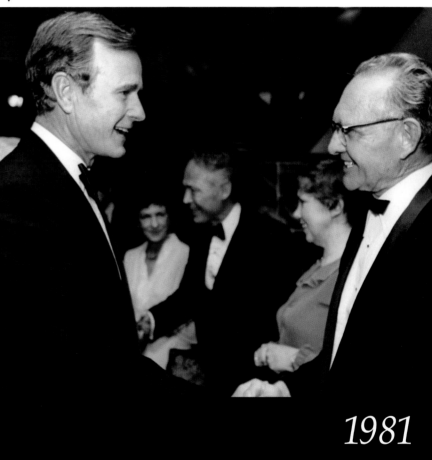

1981

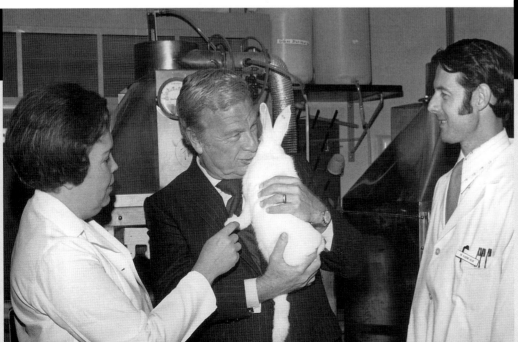

◀ Visiting in 1981, actor Eddie Albert (center) talks with microbiologists Jean Acton (L) and Eugene Heise (R), and their unidentified long-eared friend.

1981 — IBM sells its first personal computer

(L to R) Herb and Abe Brenner, Jimmy L. ▶
Simon, and Miriam Brenner mark the
establishment of the Brenner Center
for Adolescent Medicine in 1981.
Simon was chair of the Department
of Pediatrics (1974-1996).

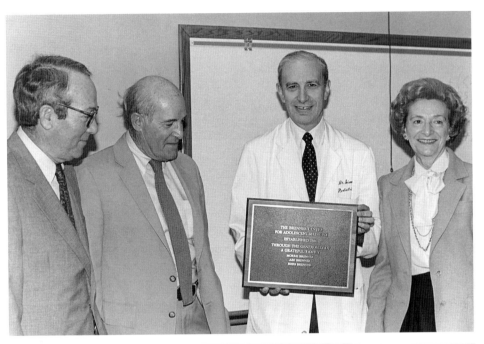

▶
Howard Gray
(L) in 1981
with Lyons Gray,
grandson of
Bowman Gray,
Sr., and currently
representative to
the N.C. House.

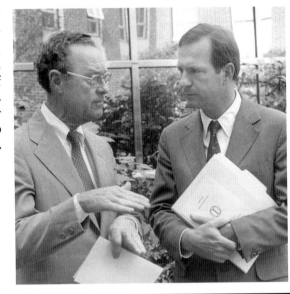

1981

*1981 — Pope John Paul II
and Ronald Reagan survive
assassination attempts*

(L to R) John Medlin, ▶
Colin Stokes, Gordon
Gray, Albert Butler,
J. Ralph Scales, Petro
Kulynych, and BobEd
Hanes outside
Watlington Hall at
the Medical Center's
40th anniversary
celebration in 1981

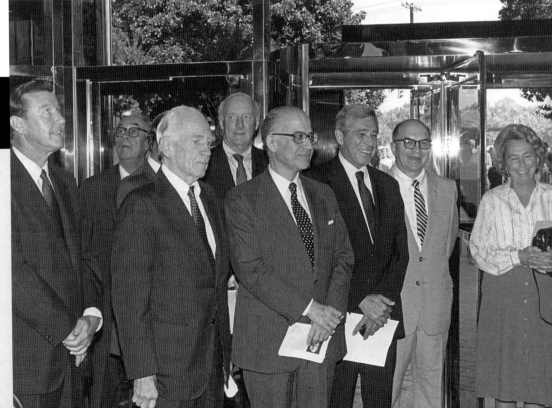

Winston-Salem attorney Leon Rice and ▶
John Watlington at Watlington Hall

Joseph E. Johnson III (R), who chaired the Department
of Medicine (1972-1985), with students during rounds
▼

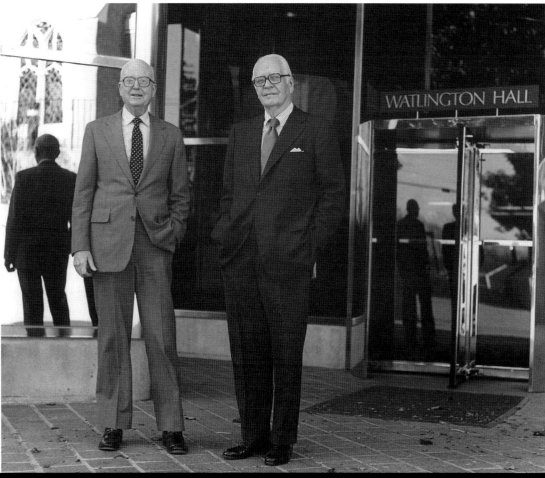

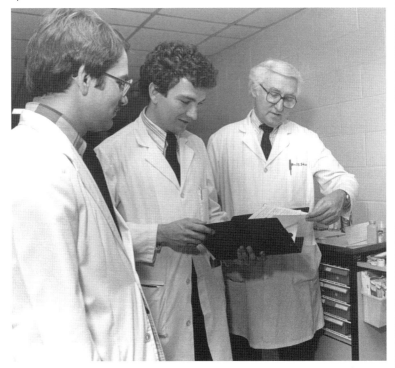

1982

Francis M. James ▶
III, chair of the
Department of
Anesthesiology
(1983-1998), in the
departmental
library

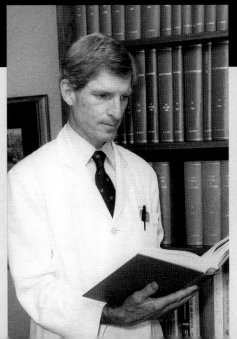

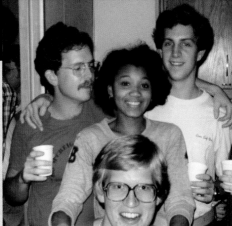

*1982 — The Vietnam War
Memorial is dedicated in
Washington, D.C.*

◀ Taking anatomy lab very seriously
are Brenda Latham-Sadler '82
(center) and (clockwise from L)
Thomas K. Mundorf '82, Brian M.
Strain '82, and John C. Tuttle '83

83

Dixie Proctor (L) and husband Richard C. Proctor '45, chair of psychiatry (1960-1985), turn heads at 1982 graduation dinner and dance ▼

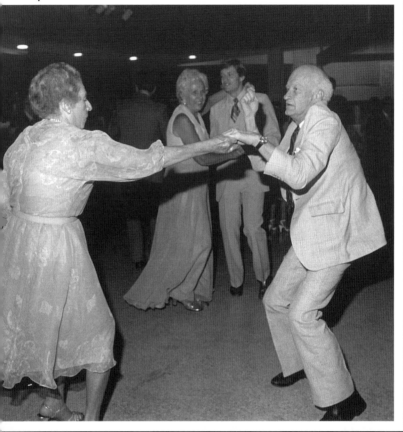

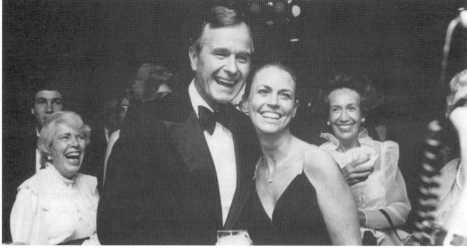

▲ Vice President George Bush (center left) with Carolyn Myers, wife of surgery chair Richard T. Myers, in 1982. In the background at left is Ruth O'Neal.

◄ Raymond C. Roy (R) in 1982 as a young member of the anesthesia faculty. Roy was appointed chairman of the Department of Anesthesiology in 1998.

1982

1982 — First artificial heart transplant

1983 — Human immunodeficiency virus (HIV) is identified and isolated

Nuclear medicine faculty: Front ► row (L to R) Nat E. Watson, Jr., James D. Ball, Robert J. Cowan, C. Douglas Maynard '59. Back row (L to R) Clara Heise, Henry Chilton, Richard J. Witcofski, Rodney C. Williams

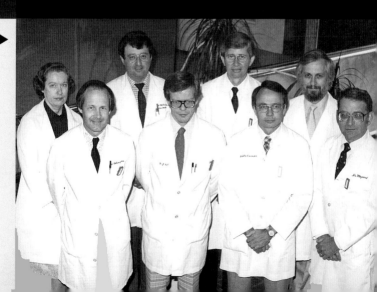

(L to R) Jesse H. Meredith, J. Wayne Meredith '78, and James N. Thompson, surgical team in a history-making 1983 case in which they constructed new stomachs and esophagi for several teenagers who accidentally drank lye. Wayne Meredith currently directs the Division of Surgical Sciences, and Jim Thompson is a former dean of the School of Medicine (1994-2001) and professor emeritus of surgical sciences-otolaryngology. Jesse Meredith also made history in 1964 by reattaching a patient's severed hand.

▼

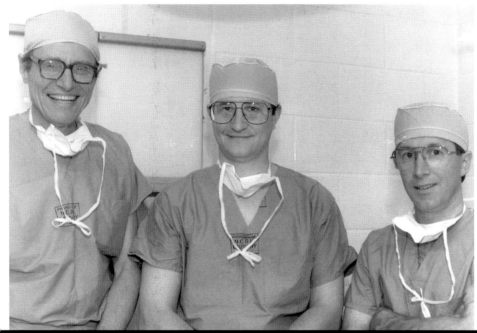

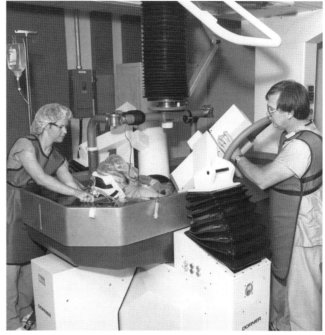

◀ Extracorporeal shock wave lithotripsy makes it possible to safely and effectively remove kidney stones without the cost, pain, and long recovery period associated with major surgery.

Halimena M. Creque '84 (L) and friend Jennie A. Smith '85

▼

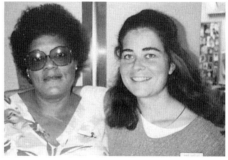

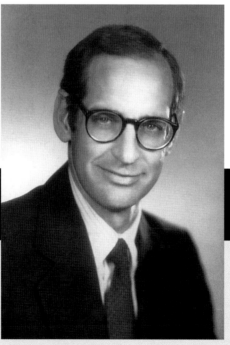

1984

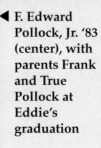

◀ F. Edward Pollock, Jr. '83 (center), with parents Frank and True Pollock at Eddie's graduation

▲

Thomas K. Hearn, Jr., in 1983, soon after he was named president of Wake Forest University

1983 — Cellular phones make their first US appearance in Chicago

George D. Rovere, orthopaedic ▶ surgeon and section head of sports medicine in 1984

Class of 1985 members feigning identical ▶ injuries: (L to R) Roy L. Alson, G. Kirk Walker, and Matthew C. Leinung

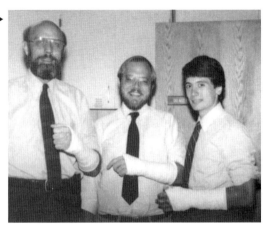

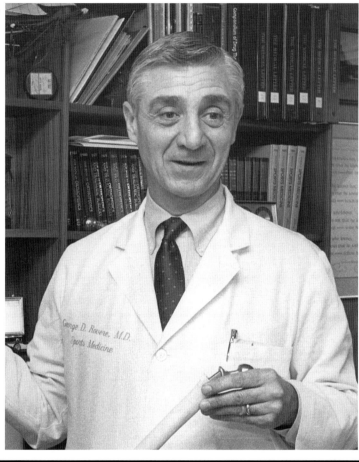

Brian W. Young ▶ '85 mellows out. He is currently a faculty member in surgical sciences-emergency medicine.

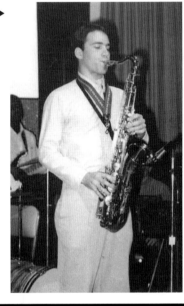

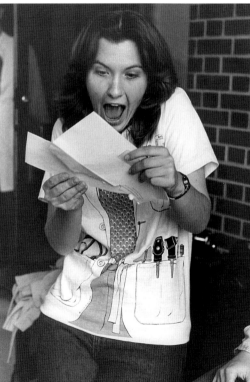

1984

Susan A. Melin '85, ▶ celebrating in her "white coat" on Match Day. She is now a member of the faculty in internal medicine-hematology and oncology.

1984 — Apple Computer releases the Macintosh personal computer

"The Surgeon General said *what*?"

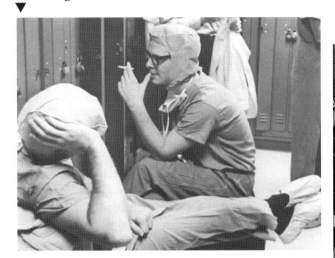

Standing on the payload simulator at Johnson Space Center in Houston, Texas, are (L to R) William R. Howard, president of Piedmont Airlines, Phillip Hutchens, professor of physiology, and Millie Hughes-Fulford, astronaut. Hutchens designed the study of weightlessness on the body's circulatory system, conducted by the Spacelab astronauts.

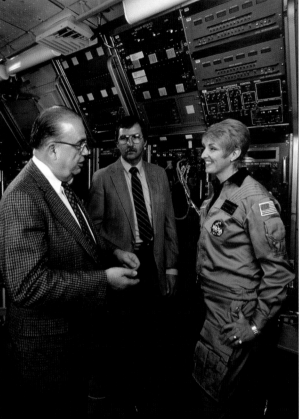

B. Moseley Waite, who chaired the Department of Biochemistry (1970-1998)

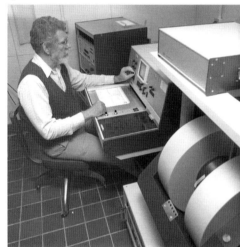

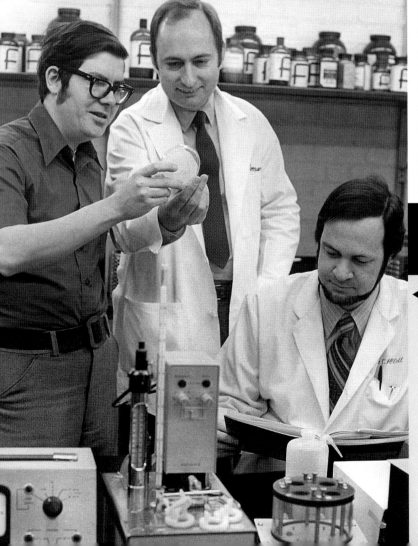

1985

◀ Larry DeChatelet of biochemistry, M. Robert Cooper '62 of medicine-hematology and oncology, and Charles E. McCall '61 of medicine-infectious diseases

1985 — Mikhail Gorbachev becomes general secretary of Communist Party in USSR. Economic and labor reforms ("glasnost") ease Cold War tension

Vardaman Buckalew, second from left, section head of nephrology and acting chair of medicine in 1985 with (L to R) Kevin M. Smith '86, [Buckalew], Gonzalo G. Fernandez '85, and Fernando Roya
▼

◄ Murray Kemp '85 (R) with wife Cathy and children Jennifer and David

1985 photo of Frederick W. Glass '50 (L), section head of emergency medicine.
▼

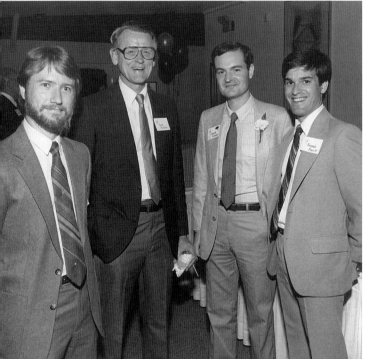

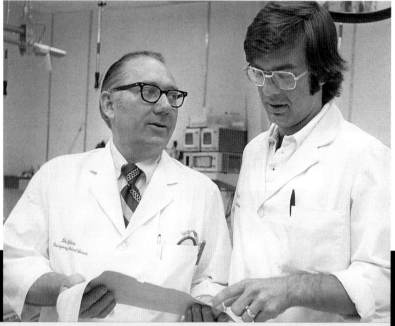

1985

1985 — John Gotti assassinates Paul Castillano to gain control of the Gambino crime family, the most powerful in New York for over a century

1985 — Sandanista Daniel Ortega becomes president of Nicaragua, prompting the US to support the Contras in their revolt

Dallas Mackey (L), director of ► the Office of Development, with J. Paul Sticht, for whom the Sticht Center on Aging and Rehabilitation was named

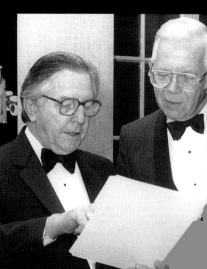

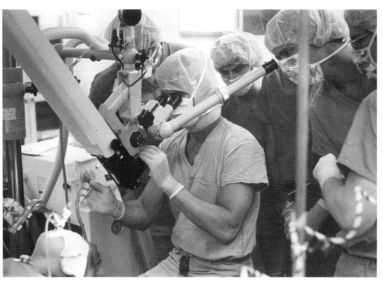

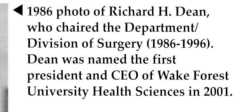 James A. Koufman performs laser surgery on patient's larynx.

Eberhard Mueller-Heubach (center), chair of the Department of Obstetrics and Gynecology (1989-2002)
▼

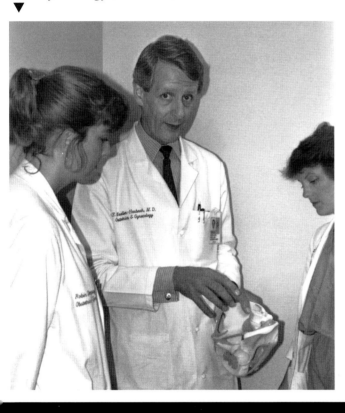

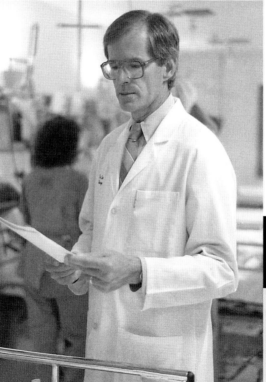

◄ 1986 photo of Richard H. Dean, who chaired the Department/ Division of Surgery (1986-1996). Dean was named the first president and CEO of Wake Forest University Health Sciences in 2001.

1986

1986 — Electronic games from Nintendo debut

1986 — Space shuttle Challenger explodes after takeoff

1986 — US bombs Libya in response to a terrorist bombing of a West Berlin disco

(L to R) J. Paul Sticht, the Sticht Center's namesake; William R. Hazzard, chair of medicine (1987-1997); and Fairfield Goodale, dean of the medical school in 1986 ▼

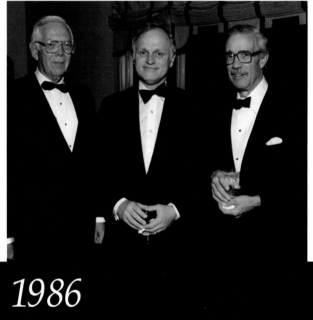

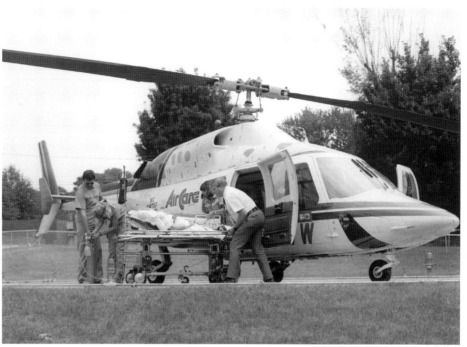

◀ The Medical Center began its AirCare emergency helicopter service in 1986.

◀ Richard Janeway (L), executive dean and vice president for health affairs, with Herb Brenner (center) and wife Ann Brenner in 1986

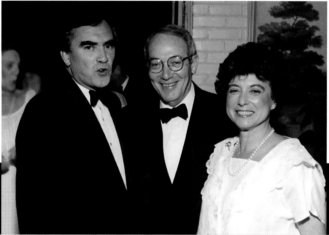

1986

1986 — Chernobyl nuclear power plant in USSR explodes, polluting the environment and killing at least 8,000

Delores Brown (R), Michael D. ▶ Sprinkle, executive director of libraries (now emeritus), and Kathy Millward, of Strategic Planning, at the 1986 Hawthorne Hill Society dinner in April 1986.

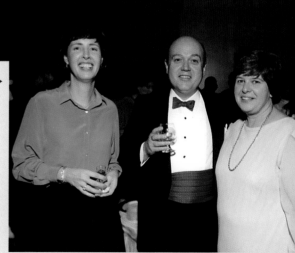

**Hospital volunteer ▶
Kathy Janeway (R), wife
of Richard Janeway**

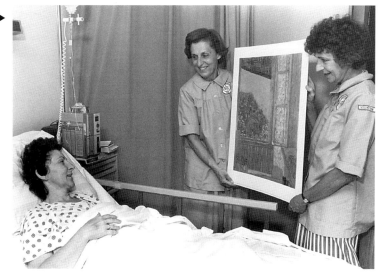

**Michael R. Lawless of pediatrics,
associate dean Nat E. Smith, and
associate dean for student affairs
Patricia L. Adams '74 don regalia
in 1986.**
▼

**Mouseketeers (L to R) Thomas R.
Davis, Francis E. DeChurch, and
James W. Stout, all members of
the class of 1986**
▼

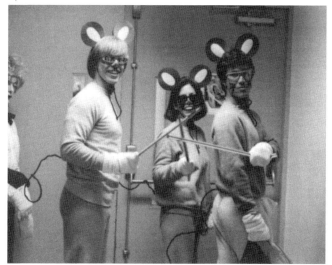

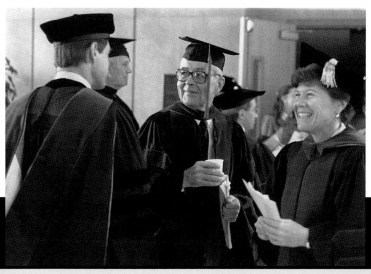

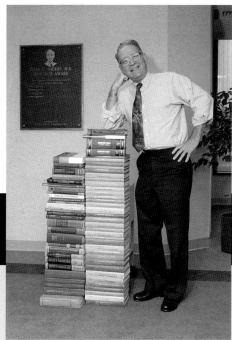

*1987 — First
microscope using
positrons instead
of electrons
developed*

**C. Douglas Maynard, 1955 ▶
graduate of Wake Forest
College and 1959 graduate of
the medical school, leans on
radiology "stacks" — books
written by the radiology
faculty. Maynard was
department chair (1977-2000)
and later acting dean of the
medical school (2001-2002).**

1987

**Presentation of Brian Piccolo ▶
check to Bowman Gray School
of Medicine. (L to R) Don
Devine, Eli Powell, co-chairs of
the Brian Piccolo Cancer Fund;
Traci Piccolo, Christy Piccolo,
Larry Hopkins, Rob Capizzi**

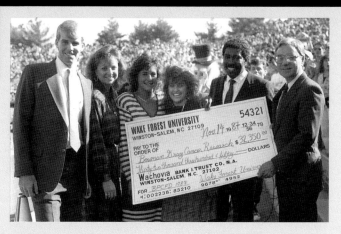

(L to R) Bobbie Greiss, Frank C. Greiss, chair of ▶ obstetrics and gynecology (1972-1989), and Joel B. Miller '74. The portrait was commissioned by the Frank Lock Society, painted by George C. Lynch, director of audio-visual resources, and presented at the Society's annual dinner in 1988. Greiss had indicated his desire to step down from the chairmanship after 16 years.

Lewis H. Nelson III '70, ▶ member of the obstetrics and gynecology faculty, in 1988. Nelson is also associate dean for medical student admissions.

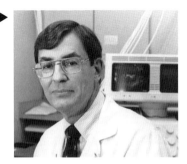

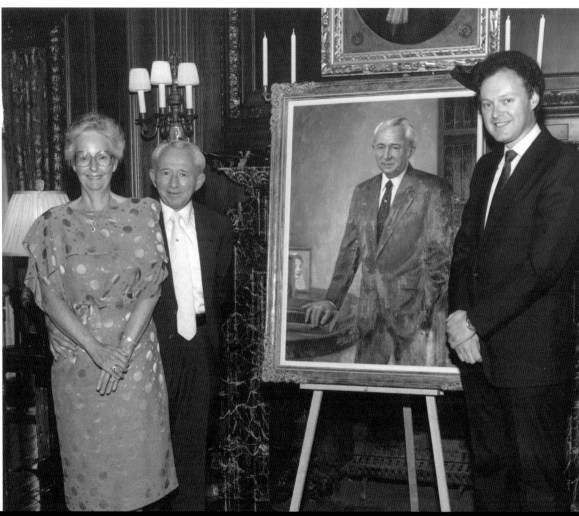

1988 photograph of ▶ Charles L. Spurr, section head of internal medicine-hematology and oncology and founding director of the Cancer Center. An anonymous patient gave $1 million to establish a professorship named in Spurr's honor.

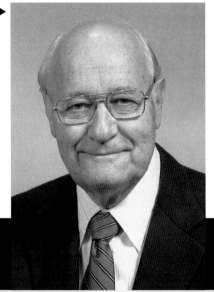

1987

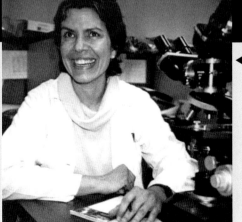

1987 — Oliver North testifies about the Iran-Contra affair

1987 — Gorbachev and Reagan sign the inter-mediate-range nuclear forces (INF) treaty to reduce each nation's nuclear stockpile

◀ Julia M. Cruz, of internal medicine–hematology and oncology and recipient of the 1987 Award for Teaching Excellence, selected by the medical school administration, academic faculty, and student body

Alvin Brodish, professor of physiology and pharmacology for 16 years, chaired the department for 14 years (1975-1989). His work in neuroendocrinology was much admired, as was his research on the effects of stress on aging.
▼

Early "MRI" ▶
from 1988
yearbook.

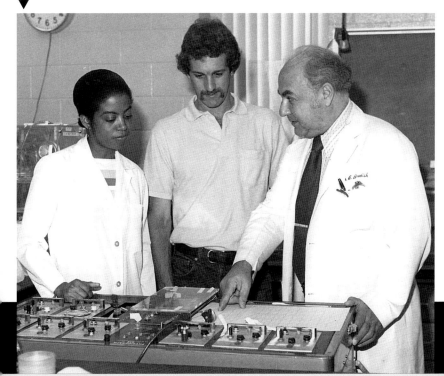

1988 — Salmon Rushdie publishes The Satanic Verses, *prompting the Muslin world to put a death warrant on Rushdie's head*

1988 — Michael Milken pioneers high-yield junk bonds to finance mergers and acquisitions – Securities and Exchange Commission investigates

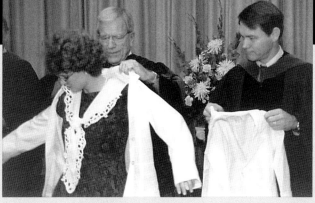

1988

◀ **Robert L. Vann '45 and Michael R. Lawless,** then deputy associate dean for student affairs, present white coats to students in 1989.

Medical Center hosts a group from our affiliate, ▶ Sun Yat-Sen University in China. Seated are Timothy C. Pennell '60 (L) and Richard Janeway (second from right); standing are Richard Heriot (second from left), Fairfield Goodale (third from right), and Richard T. Meyers (far right). Heriot was COO of North Carolina Baptist Hospital.

Clockwise from lower left: Stephen A. Mills, William Y. Tucker, A. Robert Cordell, Barry T. Hackshaw '74, and recipient of first heart transplant performed at the Medical Center, in 1988

▼

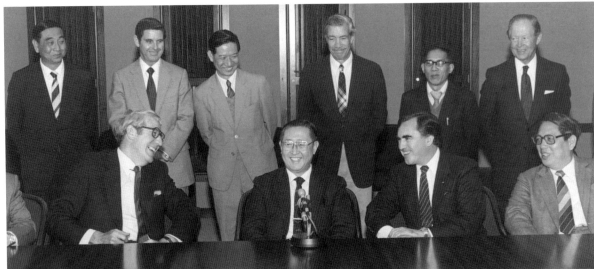

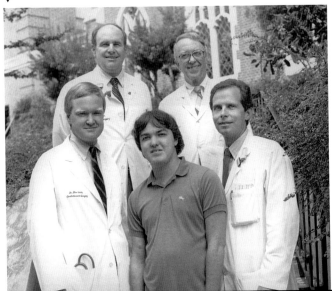

1988

1988 — Vice President George Bush wins the presidential election, defeating Massachusetts governor Michael Dukakis

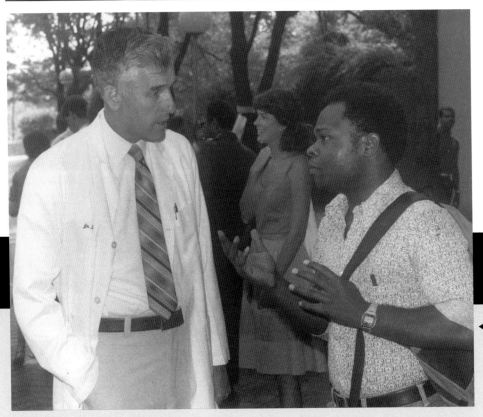

◀ John D. Tolmie (L), anesthesia faculty member and associate dean for student affairs in 1988

94

Pediatrics faculty member Richard B. Patterson '55 demonstrates proper tongue extension for young patient in 1989 photo.
▼

Shigeyoshi Matsumae (L), founder and president of Tokai University in Japan, was recognized with an honorary Doctor of Laws degree at the opening convocation of Wake Forest University in September 1988. The affiliation between Tokai University and Wake Forest was formalized at that time, and Matsumae presented a trophy to Richard Janeway to be awarded each year to the medical student who best demonstrates extraordinary compassion.
▼

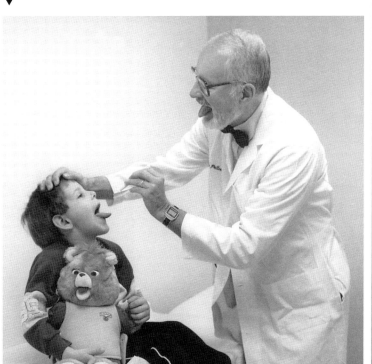

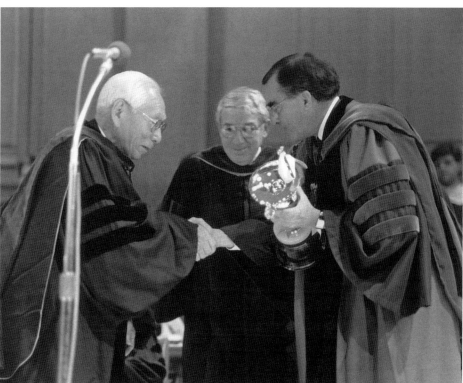

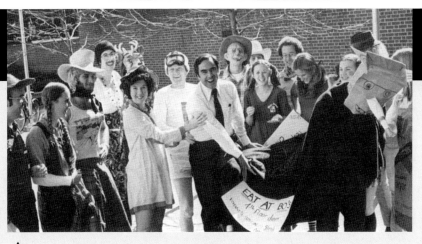

1989

1989 — Exxon Valdez runs aground in Alaska, dumping 10 million gallons of oil into Alaskan coastal waters

1989 — Dismantling of the Berlin Wall, symbol of the decades-old division between East and West, begins

1989 — Tiananmen Square massacre

▲
Students "at ease" with the dean, Richard Janeway, in 1989

Senator Al Gore, vice presidential candidate, visits ▶ the neonatal unit during an early campaign swing in 1991. Robert Enrico '91 (top center) assists.

Louis S. Kucera, professor of microbiology and immunology, is one of Wake Forest's biotechnology startup entrepreneurs.
▼

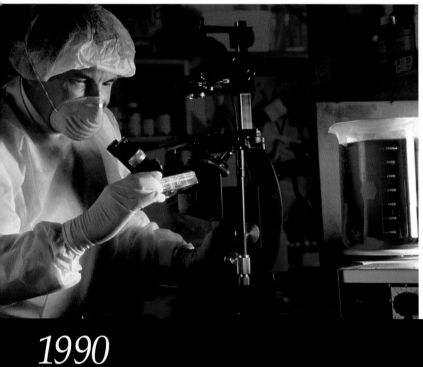

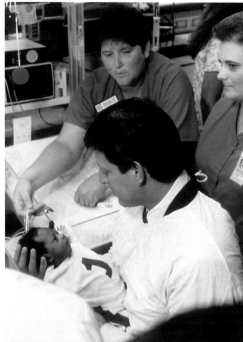

C. Boyden Gray, grandson of Bowman Gray, Sr., and White House counsel (1989-1993) for the first Bush administration, was a speaker at the Medical Center's 50th anniversary celebration in September 1991.
▼

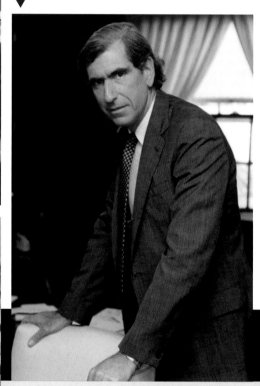

1990

1990 — Nelson Mandela is released from prison in South Africa after 27 years

1990 — Hubble Space Telescope is placed into orbit by the space shuttle Discovery

▲
Judy K. Brunso-Bechtold, professor of neurobiology and anatomy, works at an electron microscope.

1990 — Operation Desert Storm begins as US mobilizes to free Kuwait from Iraq

Students lend their ▶
support to Babcock
Auditorium in 1992.

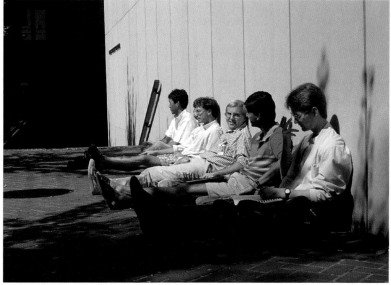

Graduation jubilation, 1992
▼

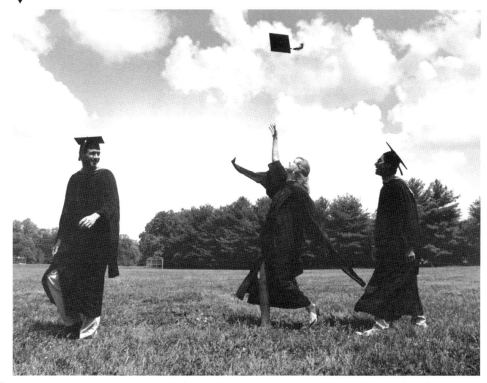

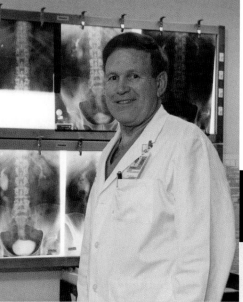

◀ David L. McCullough '64,
chair of the Department of
Urology in the Division of
Surgical Sciences since
1983, is an authority in the
treatment of prostate
abnormalities.

1991

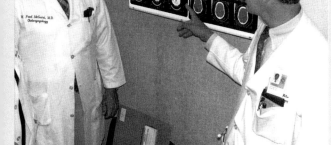

◀ Otolaryngologist W. Frederick
McGuirt '68 (L) and oncologist
Douglas R. White study cranial
images. McGuirt was named
chair of surgical sciences-
otolaryngology, in 1998.

*1990 — East and West
Germany are united as
one country for the first
time since World War II*

Administrative manager Kirk Huske (L) has her vision evaluated by an expert, Madison L. Slusher, chair of surgical sciences-ophthalmology.
▼

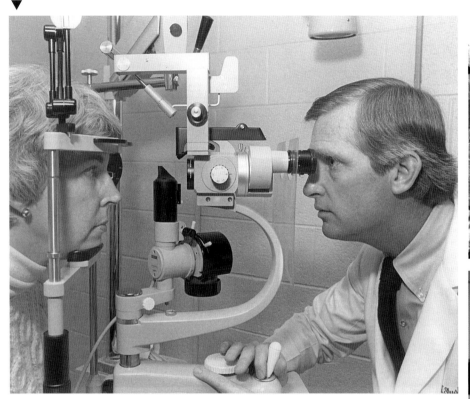

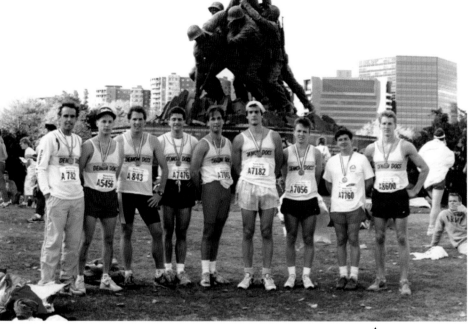

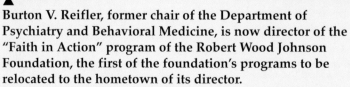

▲ 1991 Deacon Docs gather for the Marine Corps Marathon in Washington, D.C.

1991

1991 — South African apartheid laws are repealed

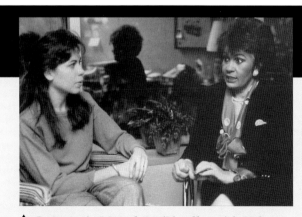

▲ C. Antonia Mattel '92 (L) talks with Velma G. Watts, director of minority affairs and assistant dean of student affairs, who was named associate professor emeritus of medical education in 2000.

▲ Burton V. Reifler, former chair of the Department of Psychiatry and Behavioral Medicine, is now director of the "Faith in Action" program of the Robert Wood Johnson Foundation, the first of the foundation's programs to be relocated to the hometown of its director.

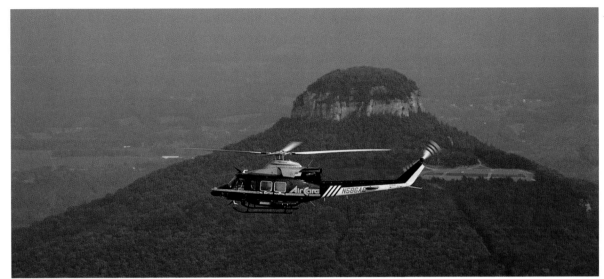

◄ An AirCare mission takes the helicopter past Pilot Mountain near Mount Airy.

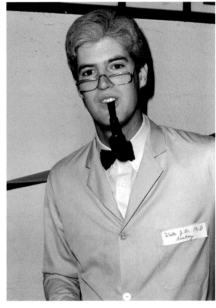

◄ M. Alan Dickens '91 impersonates a well-known professor

◄ Members of the Fishermen's Club from the classes of '92 and '93 show off their catch.

1991

▲
Class of '91 gets involved in a pyramid scheme.

1991 — The Warsaw pact is dissolved

1991 — US Senate approves nomination of Clarence Thomas to the Supreme Court, despite allegations by Anita Hill of sexual harassment

1991 — The USSR officially ceases to exist, and Boris Yeltsin becomes president of the newly reconstructed Russia

1991 — Several states, including Bosnia, Croatia, and Macedonia, declare independence from Yugoslovian President Slobodan Milosevic, prompting civil war and "ethnic cleansing"

At right, Johannes M. Boehme II of radiology demonstrates a picture archiving and communication system (PACS) for international visitors in 1992. Boehme is also associate dean for academic computing and information science.
▼

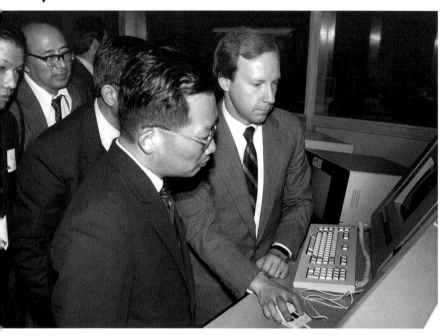

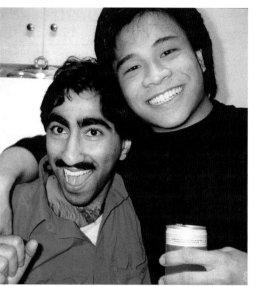

◀ Nilesh V. Dubal '92 (L) and Allisandro R. ("Andy") Castillo '92 clown around.

(L to R) James Philp of the Department of Internal Medicine chats with Wayne B. Phillip '92 and spouse.
▼

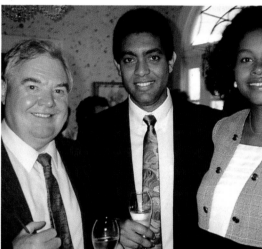

1992

1992 — *Internet society is established and 1 million members are connected to a giant network – surfing the net becomes popular*

▲
M. Madison Slusher (L) greets Richard G. Weaver in the Wake Forest University Eye Center. Weaver succeeded R. Winston Roberts as chair of ophthalmology, and Slusher succeeded Weaver.

1992 — *Bill Clinton is elected President*

Tom Davis and his wife with one of his collection of vintage planes hangared at Smith-Reynolds Airport. Davis, prominent businessman and benefactor of the medical school, was a member of the Board of Visitors and head of a major capital campaign.

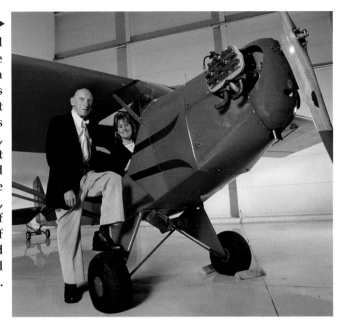

J. Paul Sticht (L), chairman of the Board of Visitors and leader of the Equation for Progress Campaign, with William R. Hazzard, chair of the Department of Internal Medicine (1986-1997), at the groundbreaking ceremony for the J. Paul Sticht Center on Aging and Rehabilitation.

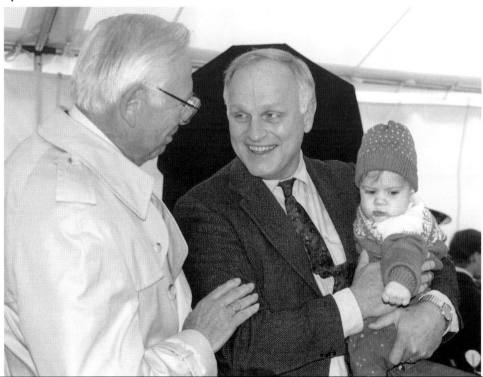

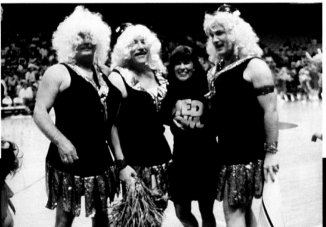

1993

1993 — A bomb explodes in a parking deck below the World Trade Center, killing six and injuring more than 1,000

▲ Med Bowl '93 pitted doctors from the Bowman Gray-Baptist Hospital Medical Center against those from Forsyth Memorial Hospital in a hard-fought basketball spectacular to benefit the Free Pharmacy of the Crisis Control Ministry. Supporting their team were the Doc-Ettes cheerleaders (L to R): Lawrence Kroovand, Howard D. Homesley, Martha Jo Copeland, and Laurence B. Givner.

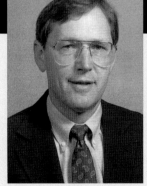

◀ Raymond S. Garrison, Jr., chair of the Department of Dentistry, succeeded Charles R. Jerge, the founding chair, in 1992. Garrison had served as acting chair since Jerge's death in December 1989.

1993 — Researchers at George Washington University successfully clone nonviable human embryos

◀ Professor of neurology William M. McKinney presents the 1993 McKinney Award of the American Society of Neuroimaging to Tan M. Pham '95.

Dental assistant Heidi M. Cook (L) and dentist Ronald K. Owens treat one of 100 children who received free dental care provided by the Department of Dentistry in 1993 at the annual children's charity dental clinic associated with the Vantage Senior Golf Tournament.
▼

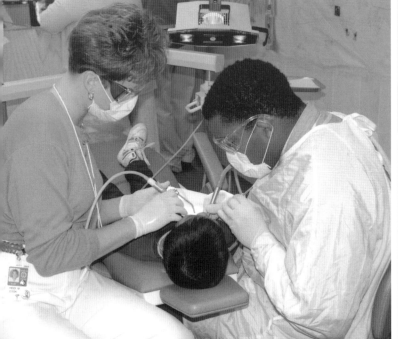

PET scan provides functional images of the human brain.
▼

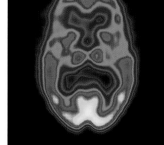

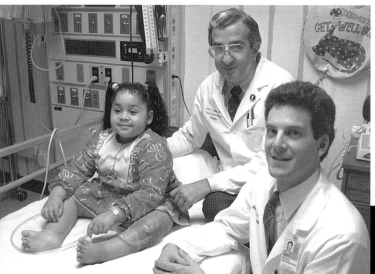

1993

1993 — Federal agents raid the Branch Davidian compound in Waco, Texas, beginning a 51-day standoff and culminating in the deaths of all members

1993 — The Holocaust Museum is dedicated in Washington, D.C.

▲
(L to R) Micka-Ala Pratt, Louis C. Argenta, and Michael J. Morykwas are shown with the prototype of the vacuum-assisted closure (VAC) wound-healing device developed by the Department of Plastic and Reconstructive Surgery.

1993 — Hubble Space Telescope is repaired

The Class of '58 Service Award was presented to Richard D. Snyder '58 on Alumni Weekend in 1994. (L to R): Katherine Davis, Richard Snyder, and Alva Snyder. Katherine Davis worked at the medical center for 48 years, first as secretary to pathology professor Herbert M. Vann '15 and then as assistant to deans Coy C. Carpenter '22 and Manson Meads.

Oncologist Hyman Muss (L) consults with a patient.

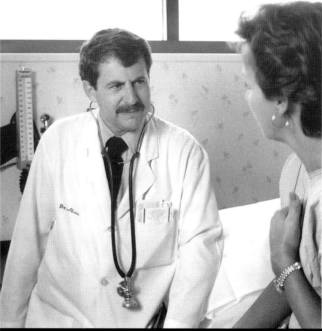

1994

Pharmacist Karen Oldes (L) ▶ and J. Kiffin Penry '55, professor of neurology, examine packets of a study medication, ca. 1992. Penry, a faculty member for 16 years, was nationally known for his work on epilepsy and was senior associate dean for research development for four years.

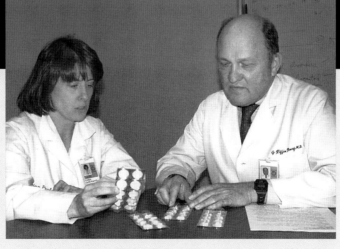

1994 — The first multiracial free elections are held in South Africa, leading to the triumph of the African National Congress and the election of Nelson Mandela as president

1994 — The Channel Tunnel (Chunnel) opens between Britain and France

Working at the viewbox, Laurence B. ("Brick") Leinbach instructs resident Christopher C. Thomas '90 in the evaluation of conventional chest radiographs. A dedicated clinician and teacher, Leinbach was a member of the radiology faculty for 38 years.

Curt D. Furberg was the first chair of the Department of Public Health Sciences (1989-1999), which evolved from the Section on Prevention/Biometry of the Department of Medicine. In 1999 he resigned that position to direct the Office of Academic Program Development.
▼

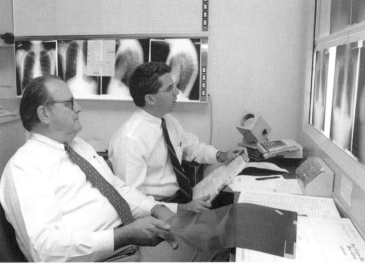

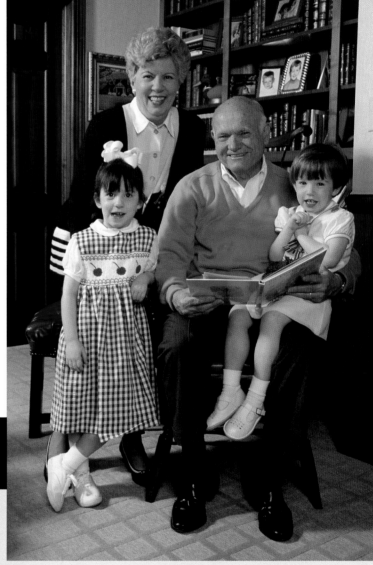

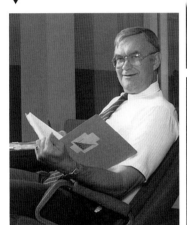

1994

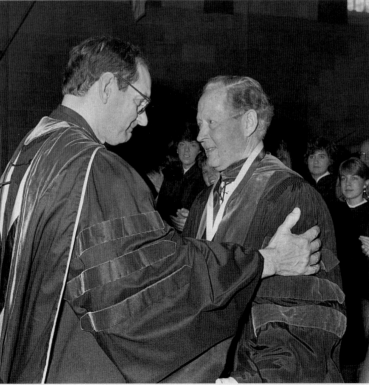

Thomas K. Hearn, Jr., ▶ president of Wake Forest University, congratulates Richard T. Myers, former chair of the Department of Surgery, on receiving the 1995 Medallion of Merit, the university's highest honor.

▲
Elizabeth (L) and A. Tab Williams, shown with their granddaughters. A major benefactor of the medical school, Tab Williams is chairman of the Board of Visitors.

Second-year ▶
medical students
wait to take an
exam in 1995.

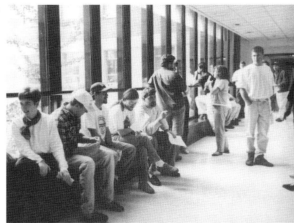

Match Day 1994: (L to R)
R. Morris Treadway, Jr.
'94; Karen M. Walker
'94; Lori O. Coe '94,
Christopher S. Hall '94
▼

Memorial honoring two AirCare crews killed in helicopter crashes. Barbara Burdette, Barry Day, and Karen Simpson died on September 23, 1986. Anthony Barbee, Karen Canada, Donna Eaton, and Michael Travison died on April 22, 1994. AirCare continues to fly as many as 950 missions per year.
▼

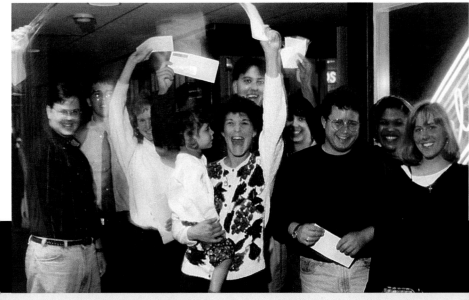

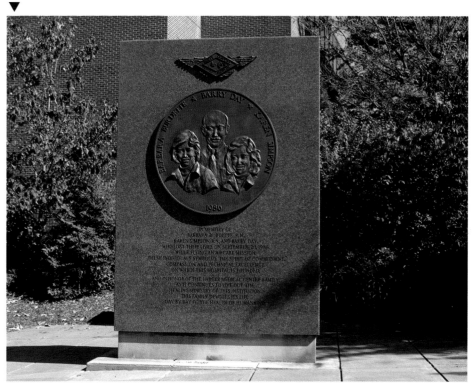

1995

1995 — A federal building in Oklahoma City, Oklahoma, is bombed and 168 people die. Timothy McVeigh, an Army veteran, is arrested and convicted

1995 — NASA spacecraft docks with a Russian space station (MIR) in a historic advance of space program

◀The Matsumae Prize for Medicine is awarded annually to the student or students who most demonstrate compassion. The trophy was presented to the school by Shigeyoshi Matsumae, founding president of Tokai University, when he received an honorary doctor of science degree from Wake Forest University in 1988.

At his retirement party in June 1996, ▶
Charles E. McCreight (L), of the
Department of Neurobiology and
Anatomy, receives heartfelt good wishes
from James N. Thompson (center), dean
of the School of Medicine (1994-2001),
and George P. Jones, chief engineer at
the medical center for many years.

June May (L), registrar and coordinator
of student services in 1995, celebrates
with Andrew J. Alexander '95 at the
graduation party.
▼

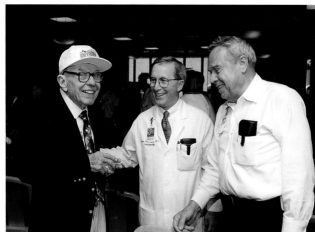

Earl W. Schwartz '74, chair of the
Department of Emergency
Medicine in the Division of
Surgical Sciences
▼

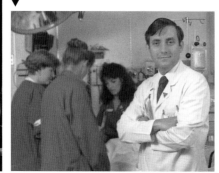

Donna S. Garrison (L),
editor/writer, reviews an
exhibit with Richard L.
Witcofski, nuclear
medicine faculty member,
interim director of the
PET Center, and longtime
chair of the Radiation
Safety Committee.
▼

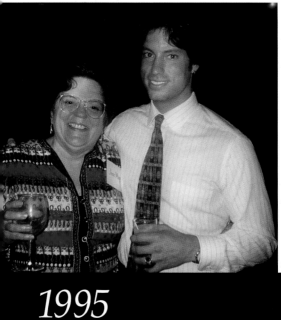

1995

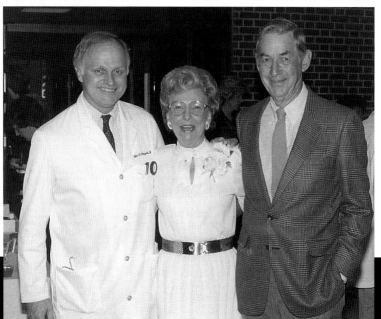

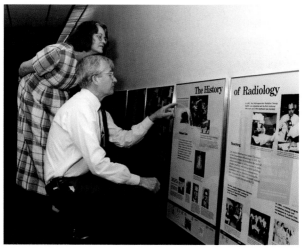

*1995 — Nation of Islam leader
Louis Farrakhan leads* Million
Man March *in Washington, D.C.*

▲
On the occasion of her retirement, Virginia Smith (center)
is surrounded by William R. Hazzard and Ernest Yount,
two chairmen of the Department of Internal Medicine.
During her 36 years at the medical school, she assisted
both Yount and Hazzard.

*1995 — Shannon Faulkner
becomes first woman to be admitted
to the previously all-male Citadel*

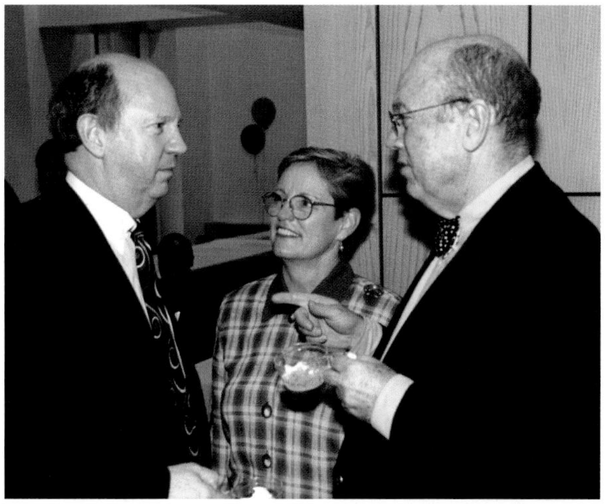

◀ **Russell E. Armistead (L), former associate dean for administrative services and vice president for health services administration, chats with Mary Lou Rose, wife of controller Bob Rose, and Michael D. Sprinkle, director of libraries.**

Department of Pediatrics chairman (1974-1996) Jimmy L. Simon (L) discusses a case with Robert A. Enrico '91, a second-year pediatrics resident.
▼

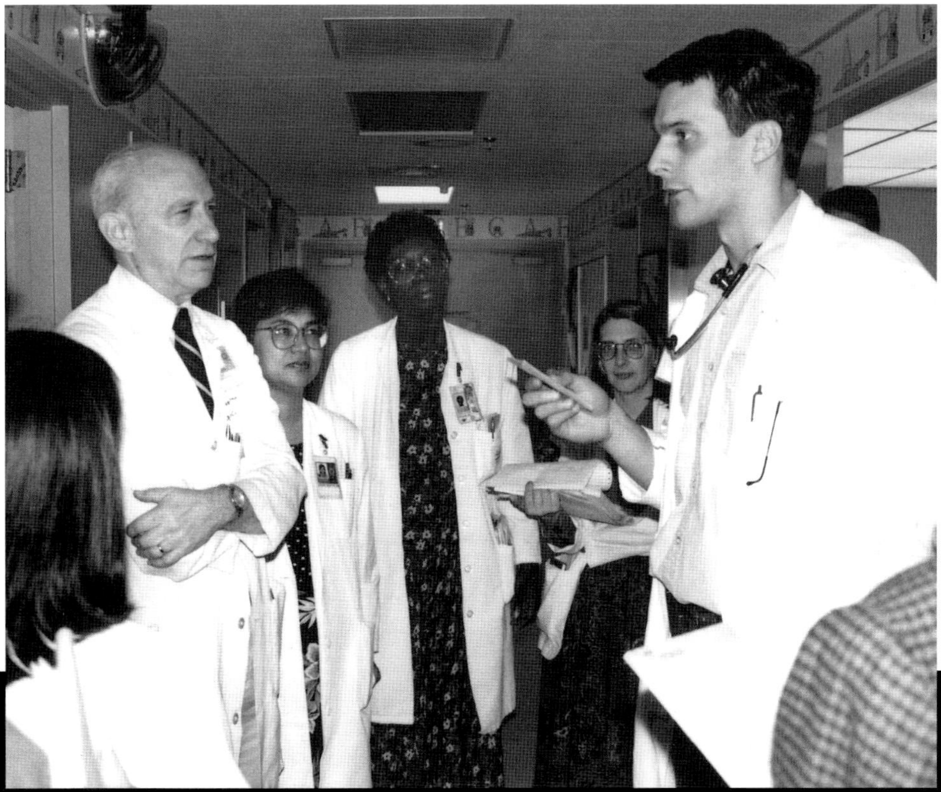

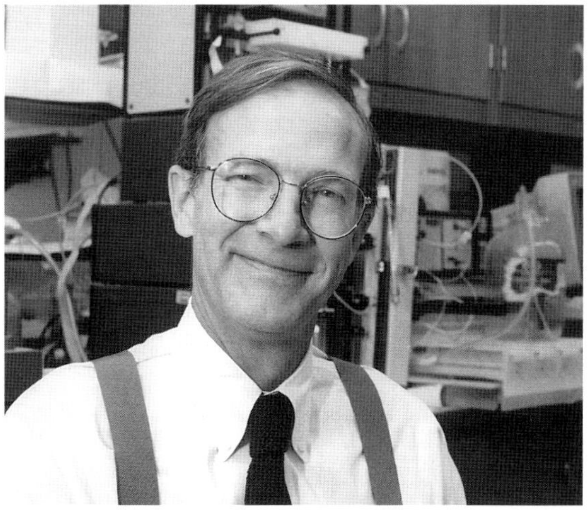

◀ **James E. Smith, chair of the Department of Physiology and Pharmacology since 1989**

1996

1995 — Israeli Prime Minister Yitzak Rabin is assassinated by a disgruntled Israeli student

1995 — O. J. Simpson is acquitted of murdering his ex-wife, Nicole, and her friend Ronald Goldman, triggering nationwide debate over US criminal justice system

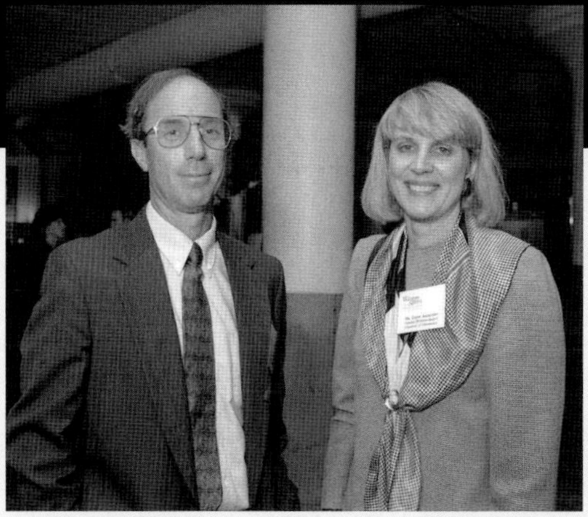

1996 — A 17-year search ends as Unabomber Theodore Kacsynski is turned in by his brother

◀ **Peter Santago II, chair of medical engineering since 1997, with Gayle Anderson, president of Winston-Salem Chamber of Commerce, at the first Expo in Albert Hall**

Milton Raben, first chair of the Department of Radiation Oncology, symbolically passes the gavel to his successor, Edward G. Shaw, who was appointed chair when Raben stepped down in 1996.
▼

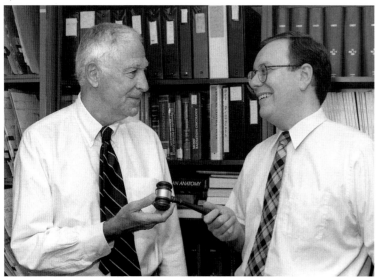

◄ Davis Memorial Chapel is reflected in the glass wall of Watlington Hall.

Thomas B. Clarkson, director of the Bowman Gray vivarium (1957-1964) and chairman of the Department of Comparative Medicine (1965-1997). With Robert W. Prichard, pathology chair, and others, Clarkson developed a strong research program in arteriosclerosis.
▼

1996

1996 — Madeleine Albright becomes first female Secretary of State

1996 — Protease inhibitors are found to dramatically reduce HIV levels in blood of infected individuals

1996 — During the 100th Olympiad in Atlanta, a bomb is detonated, killing one and injuring 111

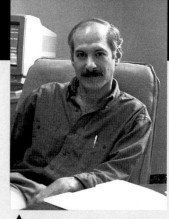

▲
Steven B. Mizel, chair of neurobiology and immunology since 1985

Nancy C. Cox, assistant to Richard ▶
Janeway, vice president for health
affairs, at the dedication of the Richard
Janeway Clinical Sciences Tower, in 1997

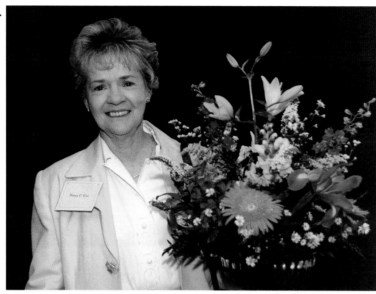

Studying a radiograph are (L)
Lisa Schwartz and Carolyn R.
Ferree of the Department of
Radiation Oncology. Ferree, an
authority on the treatment of
breast cancer and on breast
conservation, is a past
president of the North Carolina
Medical Society.
▼

1997 graduate Christopher S.
Whang and family
▼

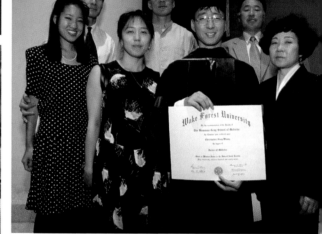

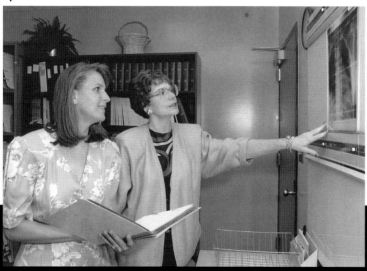

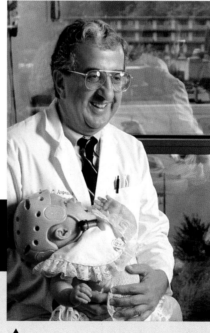

1997

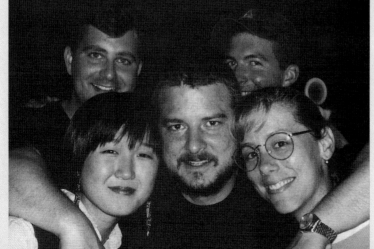

*1997 — NASA probe
Pathfinder researches Mars*

▲
Louis C. Argenta, chair of Plastic
and Reconstructive Surgery,
receives an appreciative look
from a young patient.

◀ Class of 1997 (front row, L to R) H. Linda Lee,
Kenneth O. Price, and unidentified; (back row, L to R)
Mark K. Jordan and Daryl A. Rosenbaum

109

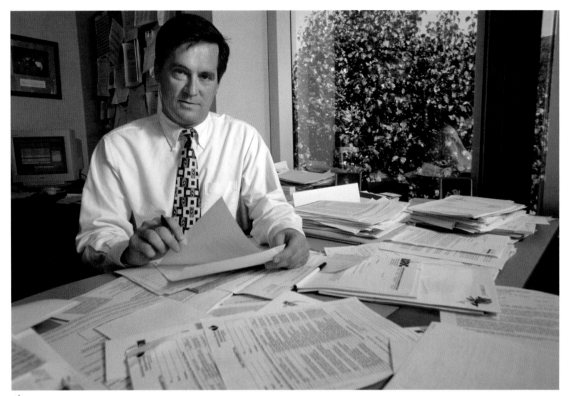

▲
Gregory L. Burke, chair of the Department of Public Health Sciences, succeeded Curt D. Furberg (1989-1999).

Recipients of the 1997 Matsumae Prize for Medicine were medical students Sheri D. Campbell (L) and Suzanne E. Mitchell
▼

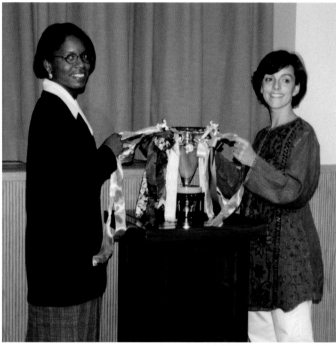

◀ **Expert anatomists Walter J. Bo (L) and Charlie McCreight**

1997

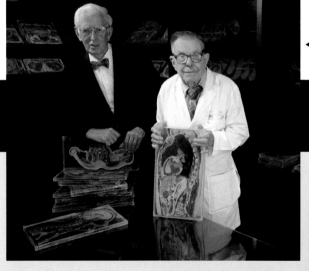

1997 — Princess Diana dies in a high-speed car wreck

1997 — America Online announces its membership has reached 10 million

Jason A. Walker '97 (L) and ▶ Britt W. Beaver '97 (R) with their dates at the Senior Dance

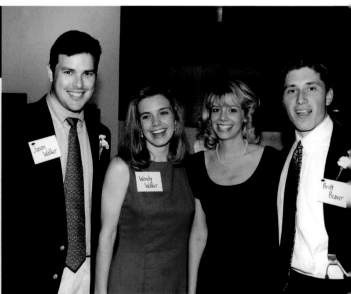

A. Robert Cordell, Howard Holt Bradshaw Professor and chair of cardiothoracic surgery (1979-1991)
▼

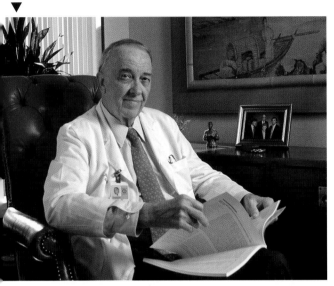

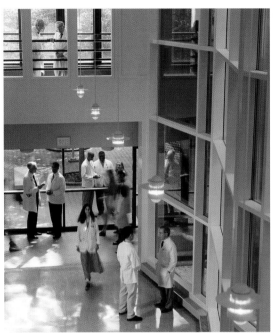

◀ Faculty and students gather in the Commons Building on Research Day 1998.

Making rounds with Frederic R. Kahl (center) are (L to R) David S.-H. Chang '99, Lauren Bliss, [Kahl], Joanna B. Lim '96, Jaspreet S. Sandhu '98, William D. Schweikert '99, and Dawn L. Hollins '97
▼

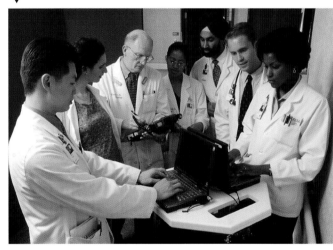

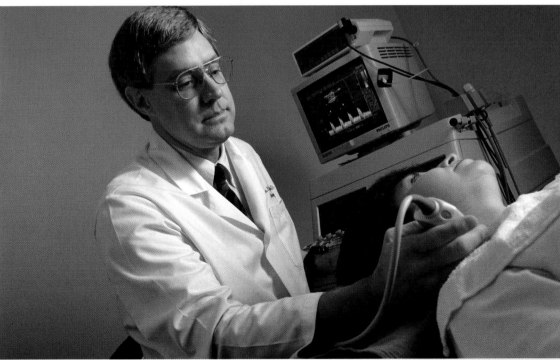

1998

1997 — Mother Theresa dies of a heart attack

1997 — Hong Kong reverts to Chinese sovereignty

◀ Charles H. Tegeler IV, professor of neurology and director of the neurosonology laboratory, examines a patient.

Glen E. Combs (L), director of the Physician Assistant Program, and
K. Patrick Ober, section head of internal medicine-endocrinology.
Ober was appointed associate dean for education in 2002.
▼

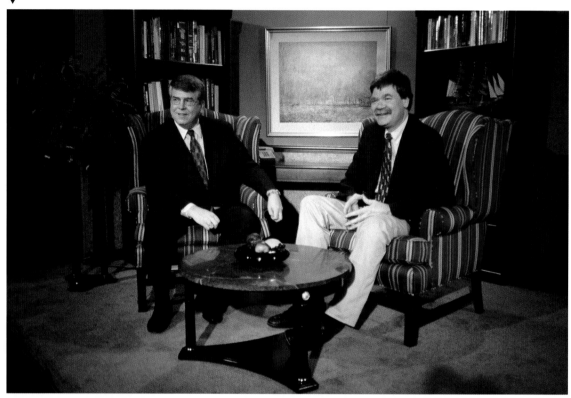

Davis Memorial Chapel in the snow
▼

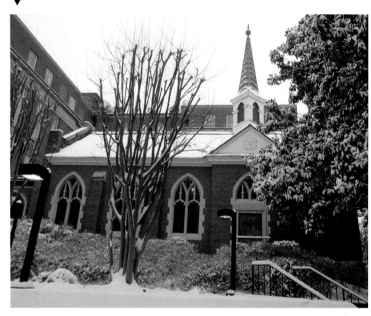

1998

*1998 — El Nino, a freak
meteorological warming
of the Pacific Ocean,
wreaks havoc on normal
weather patterns*

*1998 — Bill Clinton
becomes the second
US president to be
impeached, after the
Starr Report is released*

*1998 — Mark McGuire
breaks the all-time
single season record set
by Roger Maris in 1961
by hitting 70 homers*

**The J. Paul Sticht Center on ▶
Aging and Rehabilitation**

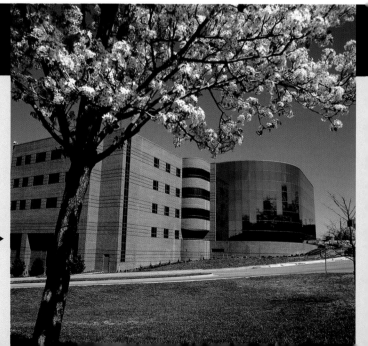

112

The Ultrasounds, male students' *a cappella* singing group (L to R) Brian S. Wang '02, Christopher R. Walters '01, Michael H. Land '02, E. Earl Maready '02, Robert P. Shafer '01, Adam G. de la Garza '02
▼

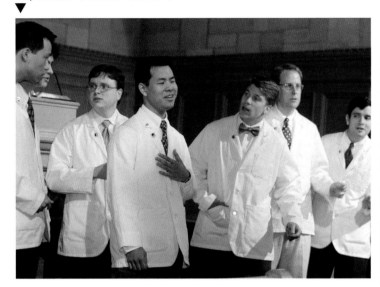

Joseph L. Jorizzo, professor and chair of the Department of Dermatology (1986-2002)
▼

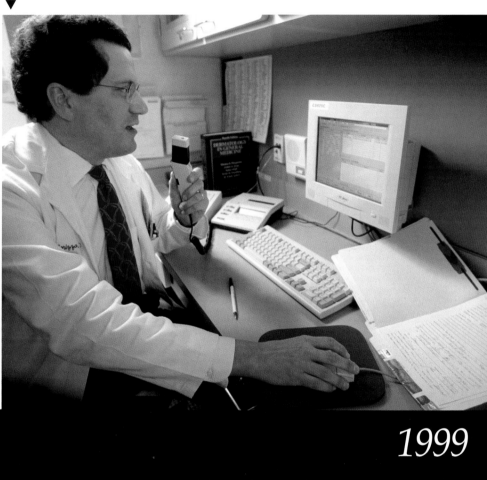

William C. Little, ▶ professor and section head of internal medicine-cardiology

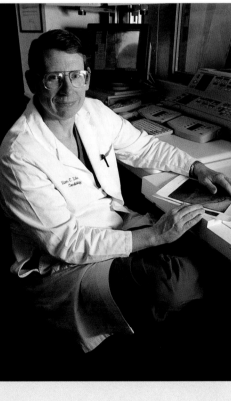

1999

1999 — Two earthquakes in less than one year devastate eastern Turkey, killing over 17,000 people

1999 — Two teenagers go on a shooting spree in a Columbine, Colorado, high school, killing 15 and wounding 23

1999 — Microsoft, computer software giant, is declared a monopoly

113

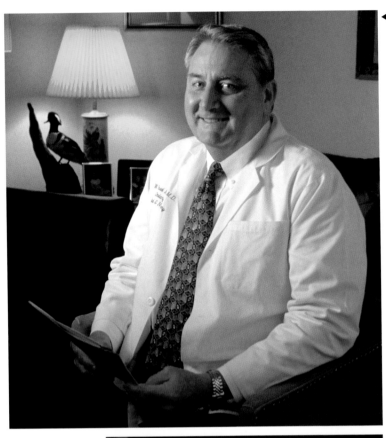

◀ W. Frederick McGuirt, Sr., professor and chair of surgical sciences-otolaryngology since 1998

William B. Lorentz, Jr. (R), pediatric nephrologist and medical director of MedCost managed care plan ▼

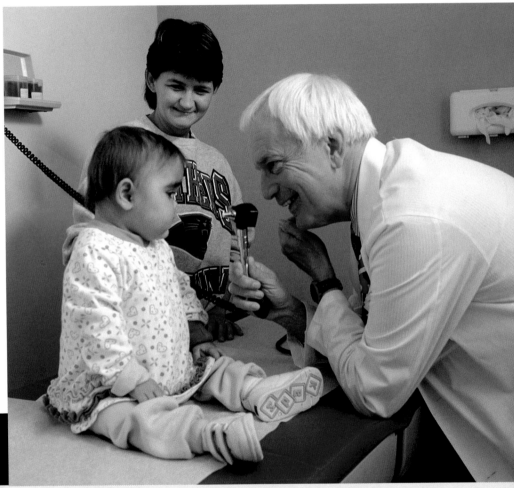

Carolyn R. Ferree (L), ▶ radiation oncologist, with department chair Edward G. Shaw

1999

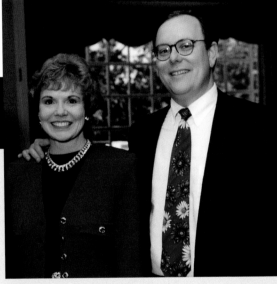

1999 — Russian president Boris Yeltsin resigns and Vladimir Putin is named as successor

1999 — John F. Kennedy, Jr., his wife Carolyn, and her sister Lauren die when Kennedy's plane crashes off the coast of Massachusetts

114

Barry E. Stein (R), chair of the Department ▶
of Neurobiology and Anatomy since 1994
and interim director of the Center for
Investigative Neuroscience

B. Todd Troost (L), chair of neurology since
1983, and David L. Kelly, Jr., professor of
surgical sciences-neurosurgery since 1978
▼

Allen D. Elster (center) instructs neuroradiology
fellows Thomas E. Underhill '94 (L) and Eric M.
Martin '94 (R). Elster later was named chair of
diagnostic radiology and director of the Division
of Radiologic Sciences, in January 2000.
▼

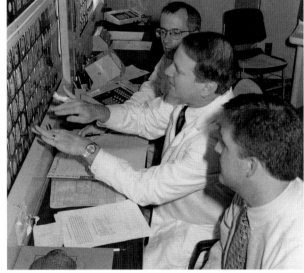

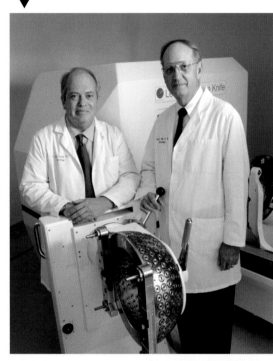

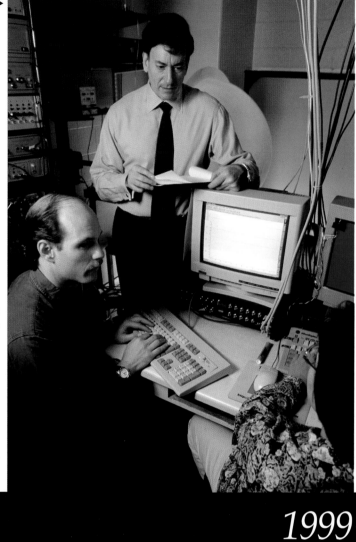

1999

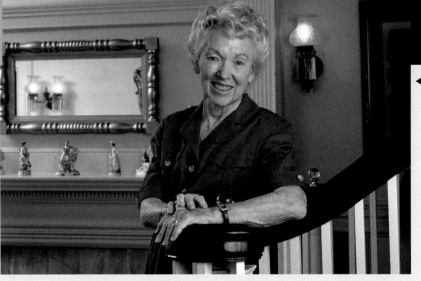

◀The first woman
to graduate from
Bowman Gray
School of Medicine
was Jean Bailey
Brooks. She and her
husband Taylor
established the
Brooks Scholarships
in Academic
Medicine

*1999 — Bill Clinton is
acquitted of impeachment
charges*

*1999 — First artificial
kidney developed using
live kidney cells*

**(L to R) Antonio Alayon, ▶
diagnostic neurology nurse-
technologist Paul Tesh, and
William M. McKinney
of neurology**

Say Ah, the women students' *a cappella*
**singing group: (L to R) Catherine A. Sipe '02,
Jessica A. Kent '02, Sharice R. Hammond '02,
Nancy S. Hagerman '01, Munira D. Siddiqui
'02, Nina I. McFarlane '01
▼**

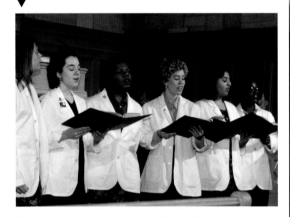

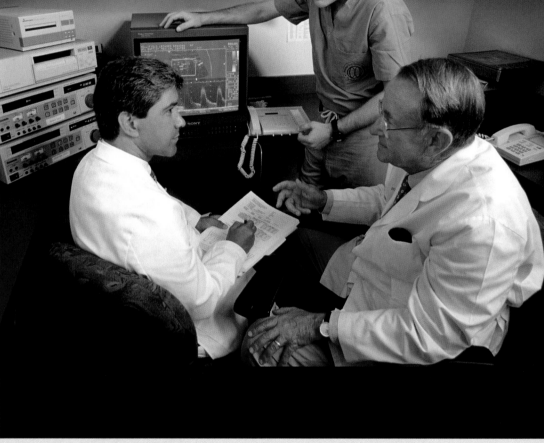

2000

**▶
Jon Abramson,
Weston M.
Kelsey Chair
of the
Department of
Pediatrics
since 1996 and
chief of the
Brenner
Children's
Hospital**

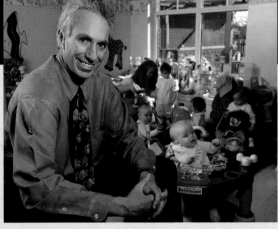

*2000 — Pope John Paul II
travels to Israel, offering
prayers and apologies for sins
against Jews by the Catholic
Church in the past*

*2000 — Human Genome Project announces
the complete mapping of the genetic code
of a human chromosome*

(L to R) Sherry and ▶
Vardaman M.
Buckalew, Jr., with
Jodi and Len B.
Preslar, Jr. Vardaman
Buckalew is chief of
professional services
(2000-present) and
professor of internal
medicine-nephrology;
Len Preslar is
president and CEO of
The North Carolina
Baptist Hospitals, Inc.
(1988-present)

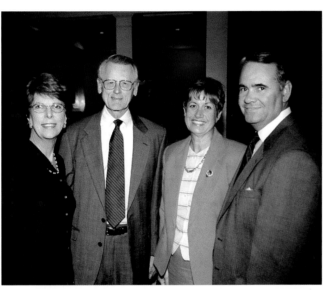

(L to R) Neurologist James F. Toole, neurosurgeon David L.
Kelly, Jr., Sarah Kelly, and cardiologist Henry S. Miller
▼

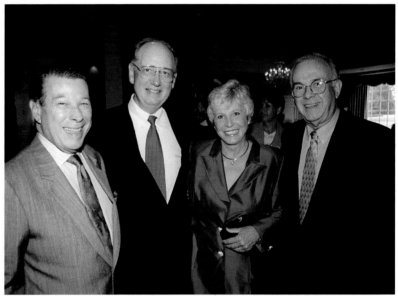

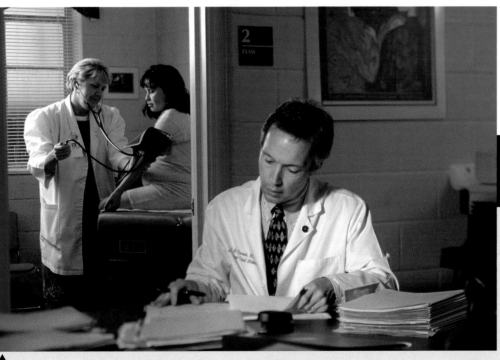

▲
J. Mac Ernest III, acting chair of the Department of Obstetrics and
Gynecology (2002), is also assistant dean for student services.

2000

*2000 — Former Yugoslav
President Slobodan Milosevic
steps down; he is arrested and
tried for war crimes by an
international tribunal*

*2000 — Hillary Rodham
Clinton becomes the first
First Lady to be elected to
public office*

Physician assistant students relax
outside entrance to school.
▼

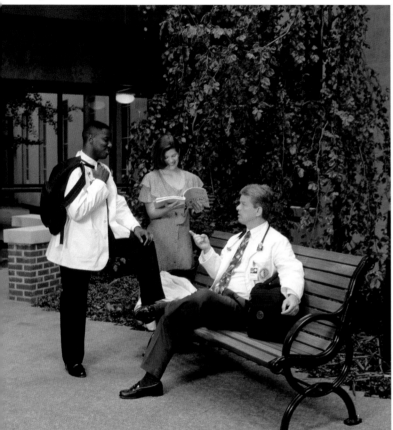

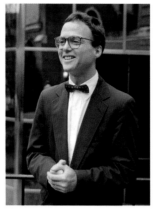

◄ Cam E. Enarson, former associate dean for medical education,
has faculty appointments in the departments of anesthesiology
and public health sciences. Enarson was named senior associate
dean of the medical school in 2002.

Richard H. Dean, former director of the Division of Surgical
Sciences (1989-1997), was more recently senior vice president
for health affairs of Wake Forest University. In 2001 he
became president and CEO of the newly incorporated Wake
Forest University Health Sciences.
▼

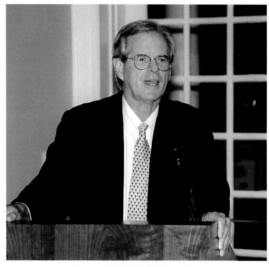

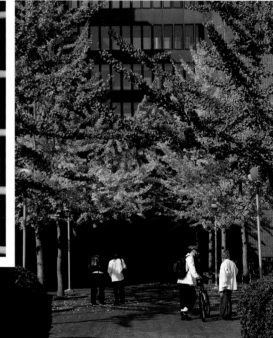

2000

*2000 — Y2K arrives
uneventfully*

*2000 — George W. Bush is declared the
winner of the US presidential election, after
losing the popular vote but winning the
electoral vote. The Supreme Court votes
5-4 not to intervene in the recount*

*2000 — India endures its worst
drought in 100 years, then
becomes threatened by monsoon
rains months later, affecting
some 130 million people*

▲
**Students enter the
medical school
through Alumni
Plaza, which was
completed in 1970
and has recently
been refurbished.**

The Downtown Health Plaza, which opened in 2001 ▼

Taking to the links are the foursome of (L to R) Heather Powers '00, S. Patrick Whalen '00, S. Taylor Jarell '00, and an unidentified golfer. ▼

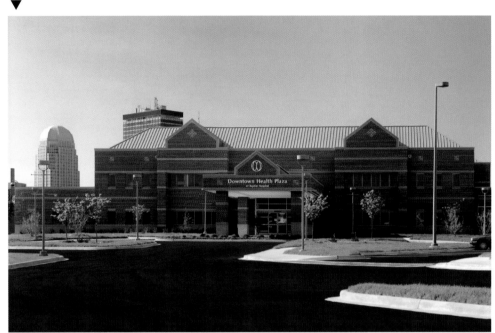

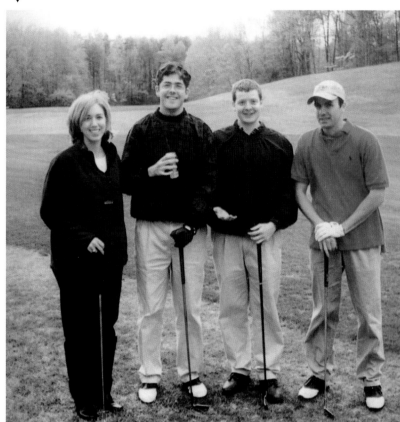

Teletubbies (L to R) ▶ L. David Martin '00 (Tinky Winky), (Dipsy), and David D. Gilbert '00 (Laa-Laa)

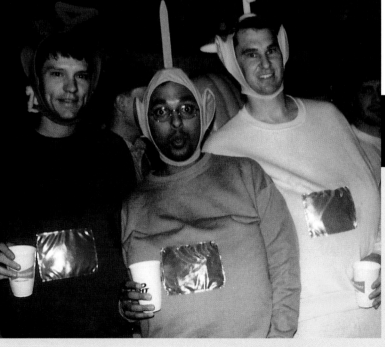

2000

2000 — Nasdaq, technology-heavy stock index, declines 39 percent over the year, the worst one-year slide in its history

2000 — Charles M. Schultz, creator of the classic comic strip Peanuts, dies at age 77 from cancer.

Clown and friend, both
unidentified, in 2001
▼

Wake Forest medical
students keep "cool"
in creative ways.
▼

Downtown Research Park, in 2001
▼

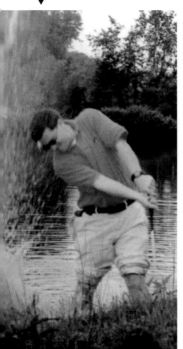

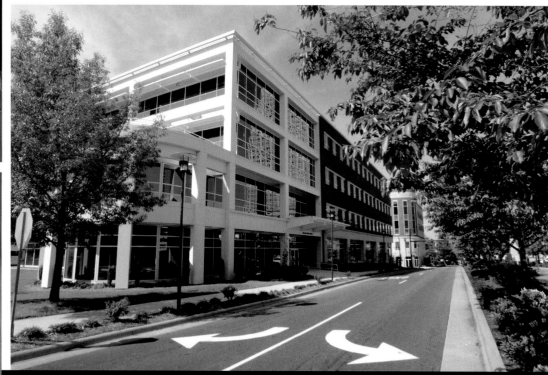

2001

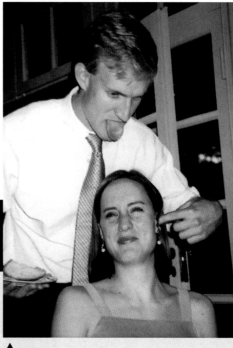

▲
Temperature check or "wet willie"?
Only Matthew J. Carter '01 knows.

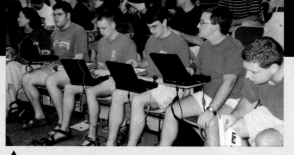

▲
State-of-the-art laptop computers are
issued to all first-year students to optimize
networking and ensure equal access to
educational materials.

*2001 — NASCAR icon
Dale Earnhardt is killed in
a collision on the final lap
of the Daytona 500*

B. Todd Troost, chair of neurology since 1983, administers
Botox therapy to treat a migraine headache.
▼

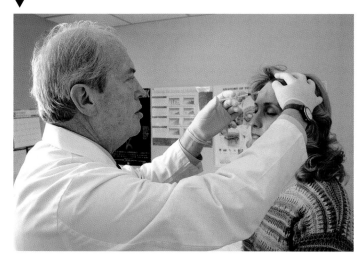

"Bo"-tied supporters joined anatomy professor Walter J. Bo when he was
honored with the 2001 AAMC AOA Robert J. Glaser Distinguished Teaching
Award. Attending the ceremony were (L to R) C. Douglas Maynard '59, Cam E.
Enarson, Walter J. Bo, Joanne Ruhland, Michael P. Lischke, and Michael J. Poston.
▼

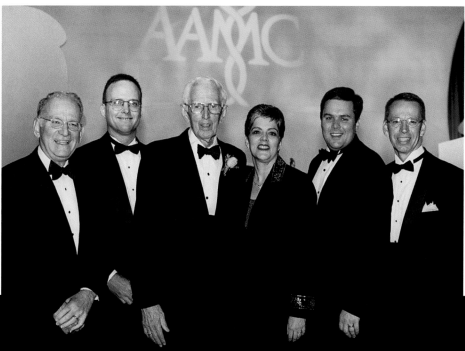

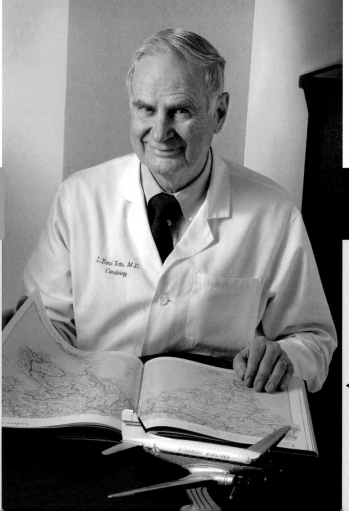

2001

*2001 — A US Navy spy plane collides
with a Chinese fighter plane, killing the
Chinese pilot and forcing the US pilot to
make an emergency landing on China's
Hainan Island*

*2001 — President Bush announces he will
allow federal funding of research on the 60
existing stem cell lines already derived
from human embryos*

◄ L. Earl Watts '57, professor of internal
medicine–cardiology, has been a member
of the Wake Forest faculty since 1965.

121

2001 Deacons on Parade (front row, L to R) Suzanne Koziol '04, John S. Tipton '04; (back row, L to R) Lisa A. Goldstein '04, Dean James N. Thompson, M. Benjamin Hopkins '04, J. Kent Ellington '04, and Wesley K. Lew '04
▼

Angela N. Bartley '03 ▶ with parents at white coat ceremony

2001 Vera I. Onyenorah '00 (L) and Adiam Haileleul '00
▼

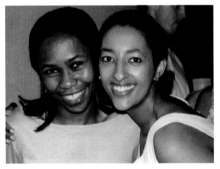

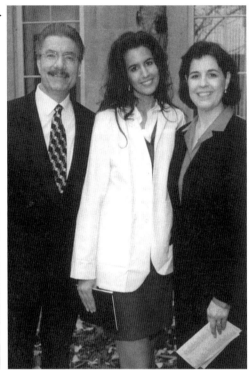

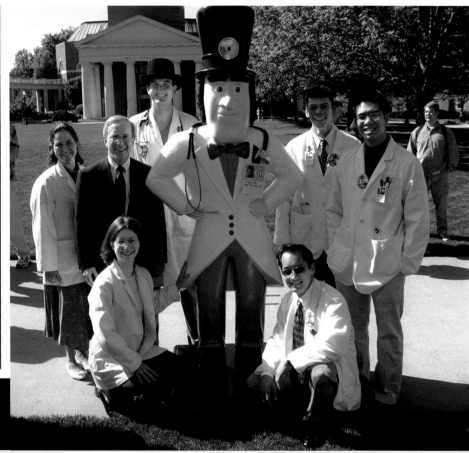

2001

2001 — Irish Republican Army announces a plan to dismantle its weapons arsenal, clearing a huge obstacle in Northern Ireland peace process

2001 — On September 11 two hijacked 757 airliners slam into the World Trade Center's twin towers, killing several thousand and causing the collapse of the towers; moments later, a third hijacked airliner smashes into the Pentagon and a fourth plane crashes in a field near Pittsburgh

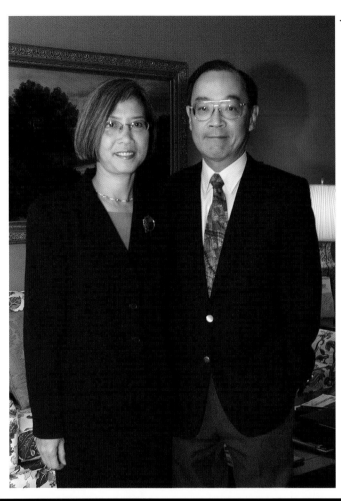

◀ Mona Wu (L) with husband Wallace C. Wu, who was chair of gastroenterology and medical director of Wake Forest University Physicians before his retirement. The couple recently pledged a major gift to the medical school.

2001 MR imaging. The medical center was the first in the state to install an MR imaging system and continues to be a leader in this diagnostic technique. ▼

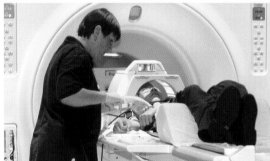

Research deans Jay Moskowitz (L), formerly senior associate dean for research, and Lawrence Smith, associate dean for research ▼

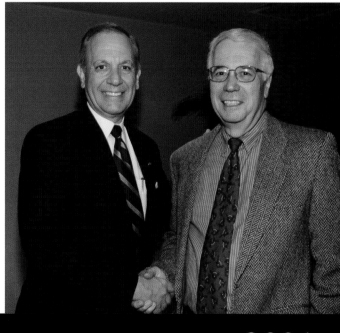

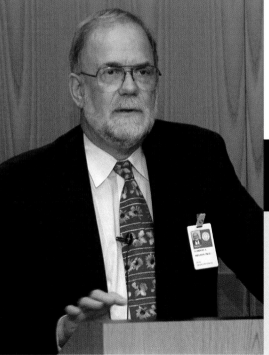

2001

Gordon A. Melson, ▶ dean of the Graduate School of Arts and Sciences since 1991

2001 — Investigators discover letters containing powdered anthrax mailed to major media outlets as well as government officials

123

James E. Smith, chair of the Department of Physiology and Pharmacology since 1989, and associate dean for research since early 2002 ◄

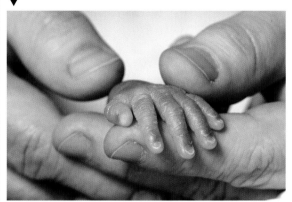

In good hands ▼

Timothy C. Pennell '60 reassures patient while making rounds with students and residents ▼

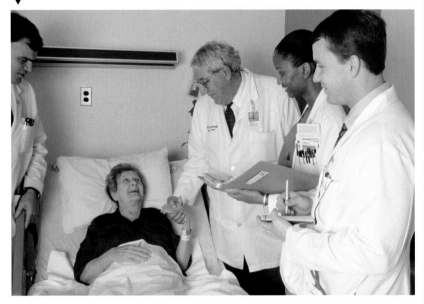

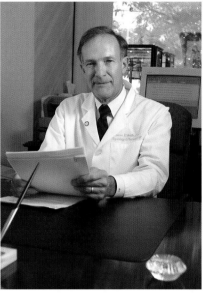

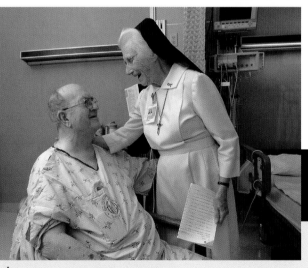

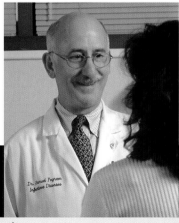

2001

2001 — Responding to an energy crisis in the state of California, Governor Gray Davis signs a $10-million bond that enables him to buy electric power and resell it to the state's two largest utilities

▲
Sister Dennis (R) is a welcome source of comfort on her frequent visits with patients throughout the hospital.

▲
P. Samuel Pegram '70, authority on infectious diseases, in 2001

"Bits" of information. Students gain access to all curriculum materials through the academic web servers. Here, students follow the professor's presentation on their university-issued computers.
▼

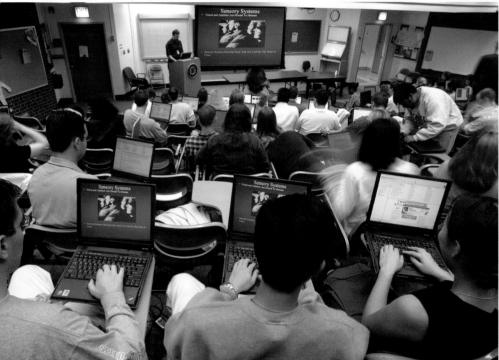

Francis M. James III, professor emeritus and former chair of anesthesiology (1983-1998) and former associate dean for graduate medical education (1998-2000)
▼

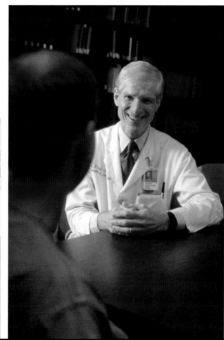

Dorothy Carpenter, widow of the former dean for whom the Coy C. Carpenter Library is named. The library's Dorothy Carpenter Medical Archives were named in her honor.
▼

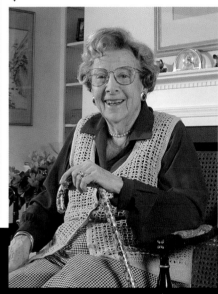

Maurice Briggs (R) of Pastoral ▶ Care talks with patient in Davis Memorial Chapel

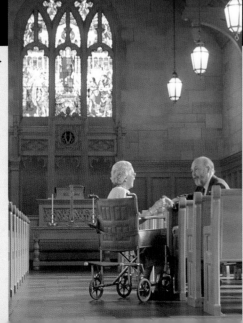

2001

2001 — After repeated warnings to the Taliban, a multinational coalition led by the United States begins a bombing campaign

An informal reading area near the circulation
desk in the Coy C. Carpenter Library
▼

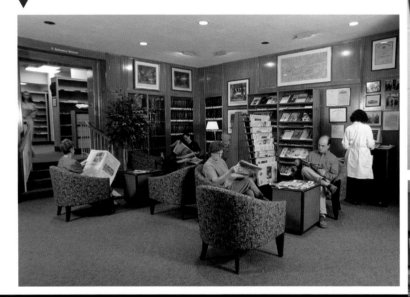

◀ Parallel curriculum
students getting
hands-on experience
with patients

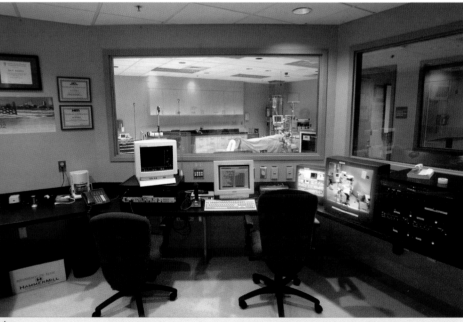

2001

*2001 — Palestinian suicide
bombers kill 25 Israelis in a
coordinated attack in
Jerusalem and Haifa*

*2001 — US submarine
Greenville accidentally
sinks Japanese fishing boat,
killing nine*

▲
Patient simulator laboratory, supervised by Michael A. Olympio,
professor of anesthesiology, provides opportunity for realistic patient
encounters.

126

Wake Forest University ▶
School of Medicine, 2002

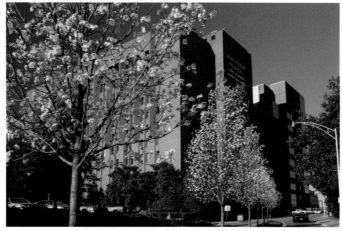

Successful matchmaking: (L to R) Amy W. Long,
Jeremy A. Long, Todd D. Lasher, Sarah L. Cartwright
picked winners and vice versa, Match Day 2002.
▼

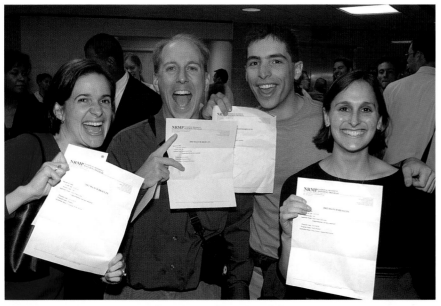

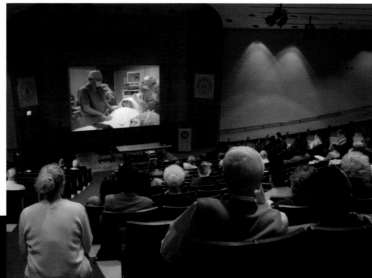

◀ The nation's
first live
Internet
broadcast of
surgery to
restore a
patient's voice,
performed
by James A.
Koufman

2002

*2002 — Energy giant Enron collapses
— the largest bankruptcy in US
corporate history*

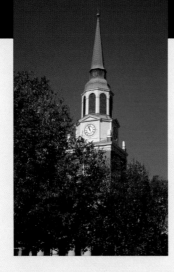

*2002 — Accounting fraud
brings down telecom leader,
WorldCom*

*2002 — US reporter David Pearl
is kidnapped and executed while
investigating an alleged terrorist's
ties to Muslim fundamentalists*

◀ The steeple of Wait Chapel on the Reynolda
Campus, in 2002. The Chapel was named in honor of
Samuel Wait, head of the Wake Forest Institute,
which opened in 1834 and was the predecessor of
Wake Forest College.

Frank M. Torti, director of the
Comprehensive Cancer Center of
Wake Forest University School of
Medicine and Charles L. Spurr
Professor and Chair of Cancer Biology
▼

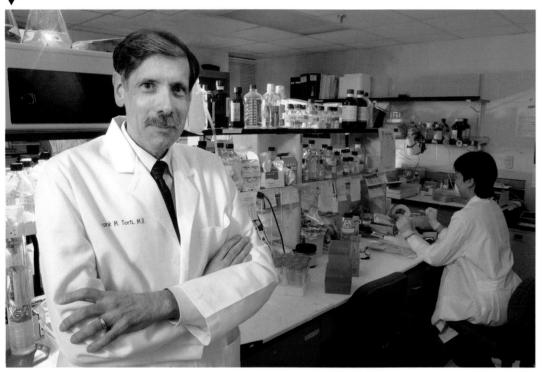

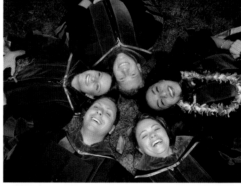

◀ Commencement 2002:
medical students
become medical
doctors. (Clockwise
from right) Laura M.
Badwan, Catherine A.
Sipe, Steven R.
Anderson, Alexandra J.
Cvijanovich, E. Earl
Maready

2002

*2002 — Firefighter
Terry Barton is charged
with setting the largest
wildfire in Colorado
history, burning
100,000 acres, destroying
25 homes, and costing
$10 million*

*2002 — Netherlands
becomes the first nation
to legalize euthanasia
for terminally
ill persons*

The new Brenner ▶
Children's Hospital,
which opened in 2002

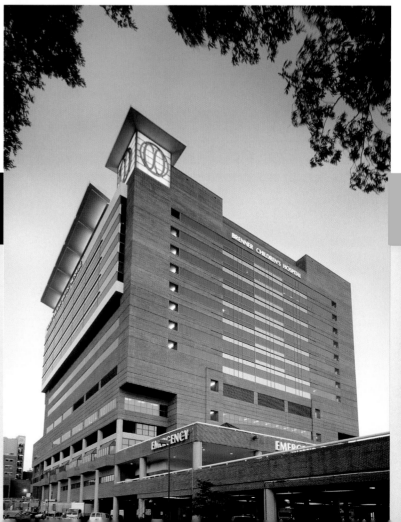

128

Aerial photograph of the Medical Center with school in foreground, 2002
▼

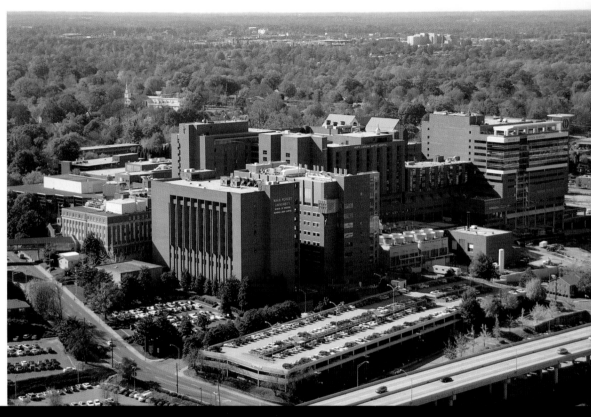

◀ Statue of Bowman Gray, Sr., benefactor whose will provided funds that were used to establish a four-year medical school in Winston-Salem. The statue occupies a permanent place in the refurbished Alumni Plaza, the primary entrance to the School of Medicine.

2002

◀ William B. Applegate, appointed dean of Wake Forest University School of Medicine and senior vice president of Wake Forest University Health Sciences in April 2002. Before becoming dean, Applegate chaired the Department of Internal Medicine (1999-2002).

2002 — After being trapped for 77 hours in a flooded mine shaft, 240 feet below ground, nine miners emerge uninjured and in good health

Class of 2006

Scott Adams
Amit Agrawal
Zewdi Asfaw
Jeanie Ashburn
CJ Atkinson
Omolara Ayanbule
Richard Barber
Yanna Beniyaminov
Jorge Betanco
Matt Birnbaum
Joel Bradley
Kent Broberg
Dory Brown
Marielle Byerly
Kevin Campos
Dan Capampangan
Emily Cartwright
B Chance
Rushir Choksi
John Clapp
William Cleaver
Todd Clevenger
Jeni Clingan
Will Corcoran
Elisabeth Curtis
Quyen Dam
Paul Davis
John Dawkins
Mario DeMarco

Dan Decker
Kurt Dotson
Jean Dozier
Gere Feltus
Blair Fennimore
Charlene Fleming
Keren Fogelfeld
Kevin Fung
Meg Gannon
Paul Garabelli
Javier Garduno
Humberto Gomez
Emily Gordon
Lane Graves
Javad Hadizadeh
Travis Harrell
Demaura Hawkins
Daryl Henshaw
Nghi Hoang
Kyle Horton
Kenneth Huber
Hesham Hussain
Carlos Isaza
LeRon Jackson
Kenesha James
Martine Jasmin
Melanie Johnson
Katie Keeney
Lauren Kenney

Drew Koch
Anita Kpodo
Sanjay Kripalani
Ronnie Laney
Nicole Lewis
John Lilley
Shau-Shau Lin
Todd Lineberry
Robert Lucas
Sarath Malepati
Peter Mamalakis
James Marino
Sean McCarthy
Ryan McKimmie
John McMullan
Patrick McVey
Tresciana Morgan
Rebecca Myer
Katie Neal
Melissa Nelson
Cathy Ngo
Rosemary Nwoko
Nwabueze Okocha
Adora Ozumba
David Paek
Matt Petrie
Nancy Pham-Thomas
Frantz Pierre
Drew Plonk

Vivian Poetter
Emily Poole
Doug Powell
Laila Rahbar
Makeecha Reed
Greg Riedlinger
Kim Rose
Michael Ross
Chris Rowley
Kristin Russo
Paul Saconn
Matthew Schindler
Haewon Shin
Arianna Shirk
Rebecca Simstein
Victoria Soo
Mike Stevenson
Chockeo Syvanthong
Amy Tackett
Michael Toscano
Susan Vear
Steve Wang
Ben Warner
Jabali Wells
Dave Werle
Scott Whitworth
Kari Yacisin
Brenna Yard

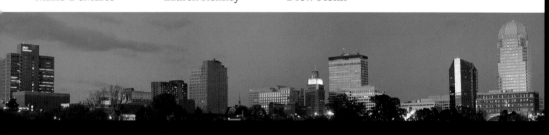

2002

As the first 100 years of medicine comes to a close, the next ▶ century looks as bright as the faces of the 2002 freshman class.

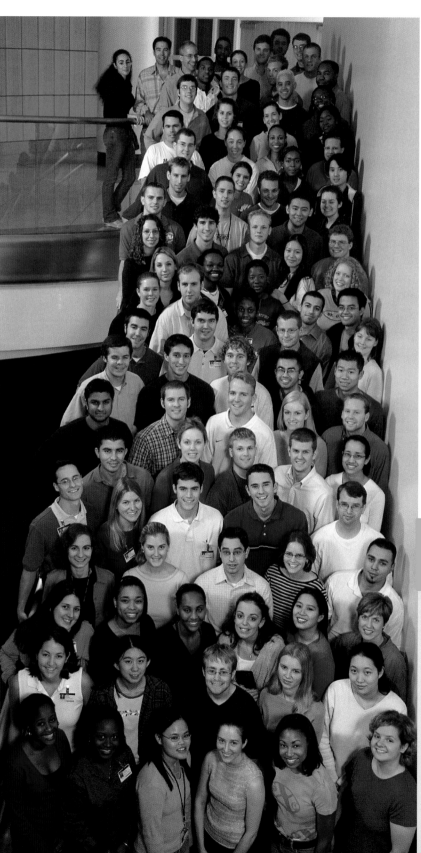

130

. . . the Promise of Tomorrow

Appendix

Academic Department Chairs 1941-2002

Anatomy (Neurobiology and Anatomy 1990 – present)

1941-1946	Herbert M. Vann, M.D.
1947-1952	Richard A. Groat, Ph.D.
1952-1958	Warren Andrew, M.D.
1958-1959	Norman M. Sulkin, Ph.D. (Interim)
1959-1975	Norman M. Sulkin, Ph.D.
1976	Walter J. Bo, Ph.D. (Interim)
1977-1994	W. Keith O'Steen, Ph.D.
1994-present	Barry E. Stein, Ph.D.

Anesthesia (Anesthesiology 1997 – present)

1967-1982	Thomas H. Irving, M.D.
1983-1998	Francis M. James III, M.D.
1998-present	Raymond C. Roy, Ph.D., M.D.

Biochemistry

1941-1961	Camillo Artom, M.D.
1961-1978	Cornelius F. Strittmatter IV, Ph.D.
1978-1998	B. Moseley Waite, Ph.D.
1999-2000	Linda C. McPhail (Interim)
2000-present	William H. Gmeiner, Ph.D.

Cancer Biology

1993-present	Frank M. Torti, M.D., M.P.H.

Community Medicine

1970-1976	Donald M. Hayes, M.D.
1976-1977	James A. Chappell, M.D. (Interim)

Comparative Medicine (combined with Pathology 1998)

1972-1996	Thomas B. Clarkson, D.V.M.
1996-1997	A. Julian "Jerry" Garvin, M.D., Ph.D. (Interim)

Dentistry

1978-1989	Charles R. Jerge, D.D.S., Ph.D.
1989-1992	Raymond S. Garrison, D.D.S., M.S. (Acting)
1992-present	Raymond S. Garrison, D.D.S., M.S.

Dermatology

1986-2002	Joseph L. Jorizzo, M.D.
2002-present	Alan B. Fleischer, Jr., M.D. (Acting)

Family and Community Medicine (Family Medicine 1974-1977)

1974-1985	Julian F. Keith, M.D.
1985-1986	D. Lawrence Camp, M.D. (Acting)
1986 - 1996	Marjorie S. Bowman, M.D.
1996-1998	David S. Jackson, M.D. (Interim)
1998-present	Michael L. Coates, M.D.

Medical Social Science and Marital Health

1975	Clark E. Vincent, Ph.D.
1976-1978	Marvin B. Sussman, Ph.D.

Medicine (Internal Medicine 1990 – present)

1941-1944	Tinsley R. Harrison, M.D.
1944-1946	George T. Harrell, Jr., M.D. (Interim)
1946-1952	George T. Harrell, Jr., M.D.
1952-1972	Ernest H. Yount, Jr., M.D.
1972-1985	Joseph E. Johnson III, M.D.
1985-1986	Vardaman M. Buckalew, M.D. (Acting)
1986-1997	William R. Hazzard, M.D.
1997-2002	William B. Applegate, M.D.
2002	Kevin P. High, M.D. (Interim)
2002-present	Thomas D. DuBose, Jr., M.D.

Microbiology and Immunology (Bacteriology 1941-1948)

1941-1946	Edward S. King, M.D.
1946-1948	McDonald Fulton, Ph.D.
1949	Dorothy M. Tuttle, Ph.D. (Interim)
1949-1953	Parker R. Beamer, M.D.
1953-1955	Dorothy M. Tuttle, Ph.D.
1955-1963	Robert L. Tuttle, M.D.
1963-1981	Quentin N. Myrvik, Ph.D.
1981-1984	Charles E. McCall, M.D. (Interim)
1984-1985	Louis S. Kucera, Ph.D.
1985-present	Steven B. Mizel, Ph.D.

Neurology

1960-1961	Martin G. Netsky, M.D.
1962-1969	James F. Toole, M.D.
1969-1970	Richard Janeway, M.D. (Interim)
1970-1983	James F. Toole, M.D.
1983-present	B. Todd Troost, M.D.

Obstetrics and Gynecology

1941-1966	Frank R. Lock, M.D.
1966-1972	Richard L. Burt, M.D.
1972-1989	Frank C. Greiss, M.D.
1989-2002	Eberhard Mueller-Heubach, M.D.
2002-present	Joseph M. Ernest III, M.D. (Acting)

Pathology

1941-1946	Coy C. Carpenter, M.D.
1946-1973	Robert P. Morehead, M.D.
1973-1995	Robert W. Prichard, M.D.
1995-1996	Marbry S. Hopkins III (Interim)
1997-present	A. Julian "Jerry" Garvin, M.D., Ph.D.

Pediatrics

1941-1950	Leroy J. Butler, M.D.
1950-1954	Robert B. Lawson, M.D.
1954-1973	Weston M. Kelsey, M.D.
1974-1996	Jimmy L. Simon, M.D.
1996-present	Jon S. Abramson, M.D.

Physiology and Pharmacology

1941-1944	Herbert S. Wells, Ph.D.
1945-1963	Harold D. Green, M.D.
1963-1973	J. Maxwell Little, Ph.D. (Pharmacology only)
1963-1972	Harold D. Green, M.D. (Physiology only)
1972-1973	N. Sheldon Skinner, M.D. (Physiology only)
1975-1989	Alvin Brodish, Ph.D.
1989-present	James E. Smith, Ph.D.

Preventive Medicine

1943-1946	George T. Harrell, Jr., M.D.
1946-1951	Thomas T. Mackie, M.D.
1951-1953	Manson Meads, M.D.
1953-1955	Lucile W. Hutaff, M.D. (Interim)
1955-1957	Manson Meads, M.D.
1957-1969	C. Nash Herndon, M.D.

Psychiatry (Neuropsychiatry 1946-1953; Psychiatry and Neurology 1953-1978; Psychiatry and Behavioral Medicine 1970-present)

1953-1956	Lloyd J. Thompson, M.D.
1957-1959	Angus C. Randolph, M.D. (Interim)
1960-1985	Richard C. Proctor, M.D.
1985-1986	Jack M. Rogers (Acting)
1986-2001	Burton V. Reifler, M.D.
2001-present	W. Vaughn McCall, M.D. (Acting)

Public Health Sciences

1989-1999	Curt D. Furberg, M.D., Ph.D.
1999	Gregory L. Burke, M.D. (Acting)
2000-present	Gregory L. Burke, M.D.

Radiation Oncology

1994-1996	Milton S. Raben, M.D.
1996-present	Edward G. Shaw, M.D.

Radiology (Division of Radiologic Sciences 1994 – present)

1941-1949	James P. Rousseau, M.D.
1950-1954	J. Robert Andrews, M.D.
1955-1977	Isadore Meschan, M.D.
1977-2000	C. Douglas Maynard, M.D. (Director, 1994-2000)
2000-present	Allen D. Elster, M.D. (Director)

Surgery (Division of Surgical Sciences 1989-present)

1941-1968	Howard H. Bradshaw, M.D.
1968-1985	Richard T. Myers, M.D.
1986-1996	Richard H. Dean, M.D. (Director, 1989-1996)
1996-2000	D. Glenn Pennington (Director)
2000-present	J. Wayne Meredith, M.D. (Director)

Brooks Scholars in Academic Medicine

This fund was established by James Taylor and Jean Bailey Brooks in 1993 to recognize outstanding young faculty members of Wake Forest University School of Medicine. Recipients at the rank of Instructor or Assistant Professor must demonstrate excellent potential and desire a career in full-time academic medicine. Financial support for chosen scholars will continue for a maximum of three years.

1994-1997	Deirdre Robinson
1998-1999	Catherine A. Rolih
1998-2001	Randolph L. Geary
1999-2001	Carolanne E. Milligan
2001-Present	Rajesh Balkrishnan
2001-Present	Gretchen A. Brenes

Medical Foundation Clinical Teaching Scholars

The purpose of this fund is to recognize and encourage excellence in clinical teaching. Scholarships are awarded annually to faculty members at the rank of Instructor or Assistant Professor.

1975-76
Dr. Stephen C. Lowder
Dr. William A. Brady

1976-77
Dr. William A. Brady
Dr. Stephen C. Lowder
Dr. Lewis H. Nelson III
Dr. Stephen W. Hebert

1977-78
Dr. Stephen C. Lowder
Dr. Stephen W. Hebert
Dr. Lewis H. Nelson III
Dr. J. M. McWhorter
Dr. Barbara K. Burton

1978-79
Dr. Barbara K. Burton
Dr. J. M. McWhorter
Dr. Lewis H. Nelson III
Dr. P. Samuel Pegram, Jr.
Dr. Joseph F. Nicastro

1979-80
Dr. Barbara K. Burton
Dr. P. Samuel Pegram, Jr.
Dr. Joseph F. Nicastro
Dr. Richard B. Urban
Dr. K. Patrick Ober

1980-81
Dr. Jimmy C. Kimball
Dr. P. Samuel Pegram, Jr.
Dr. Richard B. Urban
Dr. K. Patrick Ober
Dr. Thomas H. Hunt

1981-82
Dr. K. Patrick Ober
Dr. Thomas H. Hunt
Dr. Norman E. Adair
Dr. Charles S. Turner
Dr. Rosalind M. Vaz

1982-83
Dr. Charles S. Turner
Dr. Norman E. Adair
Dr. Joel E. Richter
Dr. Rosalind M. Vaz

1983-84
Dr. Donald E. Pittaway
Dr. Charles S. Turner
Dr. Joel E. Richter
Dr. J. Roberto Moran

1984-85
Dr. Joel E. Richter
Dr. Donald E. Pittaway
Dr. J. Roberto Moran
Dr. Julia M. Cruz
Dr. Gary J. Harpold

1985-86
Dr. J. Roberto Moran
Dr. Julia M. Cruz
Dr. Gary J. Harpold
Dr. J. Mac Ernest III
Dr. Arthur S. Foreman

Medallion of Merit

(MEDICAL SCHOOL RECIPIENTS)

The Medallion of Merit is the highest award given by Wake Forest University

1968	Camillo Artom	1990	Eben Alexander
1978	Clark Vincent	2000	Richard Janeway
1983	Manson Meads	2002	C. Douglas Maynard
1988	Richard T. Myers		

1986-87
Dr. J. Mac Ernest III
Dr. Julia M. Cruz
Dr. Arthur S. Foreman
Dr. Gary J. Harpold
Dr. Richard P. Vance

1987-88
Dr. J. Mac Ernest III
Dr. Richard P. Vance
Dr. Jonathan P. Jarow
Dr. Paul G. Colavita
Dr. Donald W. Peters

1988-89
Dr. Richard P. Vance
Dr. Jonathan P. Jarow
Dr. Donald W. Peters
Dr. Peter D. Donofrio
Dr. Mark P. Knudson

1989-90
Dr. Jonathan P. Jarow
Dr. Peter D. Donofrio
Dr. Mark P. Knudson
Dr. Kerry M. Link
Dr. Daniel H. Laszlo
Dr. Kimberly A. Sherrill

1990-91
Dr. Peter D. Donofrio
Dr. Walter J. Chwals
Dr. David M. Fitzgerald
Dr. Kerry M. Link
Dr. Daniel J. Laszlo
Dr. Kimberly A. Sherrill

1991-92
Dr. Kerry M. Link
Dr. Walter J. Chwals
Dr. David M. Fitzgerald
Dr. Jeffrey L. Deaton
Dr. Deirdre A. Herrington
Dr. Karen H. Raines

1992-93
Dr. Walter J. Chwals
Dr. David M. Fitzgerald
Dr. Jeffrey L. Deaton
Dr. Deirdre A. Herrington
Dr. Karen H. Raines
Dr. Marie F. Sharkey

1993-94
Dr. Karen H. Raines
Dr. Marie F. Sharkey
Dr. Alan B. Fleischer, Jr.
Dr. Russell Howerton
Dr. John G. Spangler
Dr. Gregory J. Davis

1994-95
Dr. John R. Absher
Dr. Gregory J. Davis
Dr. Mary Beth Fasano
Dr. Alan B. Fleischer, Jr.
Dr. Russell Howerton
Dr. John G. Spangler

1995-96
Dr. John R. Absher
Dr. J. Jeffrey Carr
Dr. Gregory J. Davis
Dr. Mary Beth Fasano
Dr. Randolph L. Geary
Dr. Amy J. McMichael

1996-97
Dr. J. Jeffrey Carr
Dr. Randolph L. Geary
Dr. Scott E. Kilpatrick
Dr. Amy J. McMichael
Dr. Catherine Anne Rolih
Dr. Marcia M. Wofford

1997-98
Dr. Scott E. Kilpatrick
Dr. Catherine A. Rolih
Dr. Marcia M. Wofford
Dr. Jamal A. Ibdah
Dr. Daniel Kennedy
Dr. Linn Parsons

1998-99
Dr. Jamal A. Ibdah
Dr. Daniel Kennedy
Dr. Linn Parsons
Dr. Doreen L. Hughes
Dr. Shelly Kreiter
Dr. Maria C. Sam

1999-2000
Dr. Joel Bruygen
Dr. Rita I. Freimanis
Dr. Doreen L. Hughes
Dr. Shashi K. Nagaraj
Dr. Maria C. Sam
Dr. David A. Zvara

2000-01
Dr. Rita I. Freimanis
Dr. Michael Hines
Dr. Richard W. Lord, Jr.
Dr. Shashi K. Nagaraj
Dr. Patrick S. Reynolds
Dr. David A. Zvara

Award for Teaching Excellence

Candidates for the award are nominated by the medical students and selected by a committee comprised of students and faculty.

1973	Robert W. Prichard	1988	P. Samuel Pegram, Jr.
1974	Robert C. McKone	1989	Joseph M. Ernest III
1975	Lawrence R. DeChatelet	1990	W. Keith O'Steen
1976	Jimmy L. Simon	1991	Edward F. Haponik
1977	N. Sheldon Skinner, Jr.	1992	James E. Peacock
1978	Harold O. Goodman	1993	K. Patrick Ober
1979	Michael A. Moore	1994	Peter B. Smith
1980	Peter B. Smith	1995	Walter J. Bo
1981	Timothy C. Pennell	1996	Elizabeth Sherertz
1982	Vardaman M. Buckalew, Jr.	1997	Jack W. Strandhoy
1983	Charles E. McCreight	1998	Michael R. Lawless
1984	K. Patrick Ober	1999	Edward F. Haponik
1985	Walter J. Bo	2000	Robert L. Bowden
1986	B. Todd Troost	2001	James E. Johnson
1987	Julia M. Cruz	2002	Lawrence B. Givner

Yearbook Dedications

1941	Edgar Estes Folk	1973	M. Robert Cooper
1942	Elliott B. Earnshaw	1974	John H. Edmonds, Jr.
1943	Henry Broadus Jones	1975	A. Sherrill Hudspeth
1944	Wingate M. Johnson	1976	Jimmy Simon
1945	Dedicated to all grads in the military	1977	N. Sheldon Skinner
1946	Howard Holt Bradshaw	1978	Paul B. Comer
1947	Herbert Moffit Vann		Robert L. Gibson
1948	Wilbur C. Thomas	1979	Lawrence R. DeChatelet
1949	No yearbook published	1980	Charles E. McCreight
1950	Robert P. "Moose" Morehead	1981	Timothy C. Pennell
1951	George T. Harrell, Jr.	1982	Ruth O'Neal
1952	Robert Lindsay McMillan	1983	Eben Alexander, Jr.
1953	Eben Alexander, Jr.	1984	Isadore Meschan
1954	Robert W. Lawson	1985	K. Patrick Ober
	Weston M. Kelsey	1986	Ronald B. Mack
1955	Robert W. Prichard	1987	Richard Thomas Myers
1956	Coy C. Carpenter		Margaret Geraldine Peavy
1957	Ernest H. Yount, Jr.	1988	Paul Samuel Pegram, Jr.
1958	Robert J. Tuttle	1989	Craig Gallanis
1959	Harold D. Green	1990	Walter John Bo
1960	Charles L. Spurr	1991	Richard Janeway
1961	Katherine Davis	1992	Timothy C. Pennell
1962	Weston M. Kelsey	1993	Charles S. Turner
1963	Camillo Artom	1994	Michael R. Lawless
1964	Isadore Meschan	1995	June G. May
1965	Robert P. Morehead	1996	Jimmy L. Simon
1966	James F. Toole	1997	K. Patrick Ober
1967	LeRoy Crandell	1998	Edward F. Haponik
1968	Donald M. Hayes	1999	Patricia L. Adams
1969	Timothy C. Pennell	2000	B. Todd Troost
1970	Earl Watts	2001	Venita Morrell
1971	Robert Prichard		Brenda Latham-Sadler
1972	Charles E. McCall	2002	James N. Thompson

MAA Presidents

Date of Service/Name/Class Year

1943-44	Louten R. Hedgpeth '31	1976	Giles L. Cloninger '54
1945-46	Bahnson Weathers '15	1977	Wayne A. Cline, Sr. '46
1947	George Oren Moss '25	1978	Livingston Johnson '51
1948	Felda Hightower '31	1979	Robert Clyde Pope '45
1949-50	Thomas William Baker '29	1980	Carey James Walton, Jr. '55
1951-52	David Russell Perry, Sr. '17	1981	Murphy F. Townsend, Jr. '61
1953	Ernest Furgurson '34	1982	Gary B. Copeland '60
1954	Eugene C. Clayton '45	1983	Dixie Lee Boney Soo '59
1955	H. Fleming Fuller '34	1984	Charles R. Duncan, Jr. '63
1956	Vernon W. Taylor '36	1985	M Frank Sohmer '52
1957	L. Randolph Doffermyre '35	1986	W. Claude Hollingsworth '59
1958	Roscoe L. Wall '10	1987	Manly Y. Brunt '48
1959	Claude A. McNeill '43	1988	Joe H. Woody '58
1960	D. E. Ward '45	1989	Robert Lee Vann '45
1961	George W. Paschal, Jr. '29	1990	Neill H. Musselwhite III '75
1962	D. Russell Perry, Jr. '46	1991	Mary Ann Taylor '60
1963	Jerome Otis Williams '46	1992	Kyle A. Young '69
1964	Hubert M. Poteat '38	1993	W. Hampton Lefler, Jr. '63
1965	Julian F. Keith, Jr. '53	1994-1995	Timothy F. Edwards '78
1966	Walton Kitchin '38	1995-1996	Howard G. Dawkins, Jr. '68
1967	W. Boyd Owen '40	1996-1997	Thomas J. Pulliam '84
1968	W. H (Joe) Freeman '44	1997-1998	Joel B. Miller '74
1969	Robert Perry Crouch '54	1998-1999	Patricia C. Farrell '87
1970	Joseph B. Alexander '47	1999-2000	George H. Wall '58
1971	Claude A. McNeill '43	2000-2001	George W. Paschal III '73
1972	Jefferson D. Beale '44	2001-2002	Sam R. Fulp '83
1973	John Wesley Nance '48	2002-2003	Thomas H. Hunt '71
1974	Jean Bailey Brooks '44		
1975	Ernest H. Stines '57		

MAA Award Recipients

DISTINGUISHED ACHIEVEMENT AWARD

1982	E. Garland Herndon, Jr., MD '46	1994	W. Claude Hollingsworth, MD '59
1986	Paul P. Griffin, MD '53	1995	W. Hampton Lefler, Jr., MD '63
1987	C. Douglas Maynard, MD '59	1996	Katherine Davis
1988	John A. Oates, Jr., MD '56	1997	Mary Ann Hampton Taylor, MD '60
1989	Joseph E. Whitley, MD '55	1998	Joe H. Woody, MD '58
1989	James G. Jones, MD '59	1999	Howard G. Dawkins, Jr., MD '68
1990	Byron G. Brogdon, MD, FHO	1999	Howard S. Wainer, MD '54
1990	J. Kiffin Penry, MD '55	2000	Max Wainer
1991	John M. Tew, Jr., MD '61	2001	John C. Whitaker, Jr.
1991	David M. Drylie, MD '56	2002	Neill Musselwhite, M.D. '75
1992	Paul D. Webster III, MD '56		
1993	Richard B. Odom, MD '63		
1994	Robert H. Shackelford, MD '47		

DISTINGUISHED FACULTY SERVICE AWARD

1988	Robert P. Morehead, MD '34
1989	Eben Alexander, Jr., MD
1989	Isadore Meschan, MD
1990	Ernest H. Young, Jr., MD
1991	Richard T. Myers, MD, FHO
1992	Charles L. Spurr, MD
1993	Emery C. Miller, MD, FHO
1994	Richard G. Weaver, MD, FHO
1995	Walter E. Bo, Ph.D.
1995	Charles E. McCreight, Ph.D.
1996	James F. Toole, MD
1996	Timothy C. Pennell, MD '60
1997	Francis M. James III, MD
1997	M. Robert Cooper, MD '62
1998	Robert N. Headley, M.D., FHO
1999	Lewis H. Nelson III, MD '70
1999	Charles E. McCall, MD '61
2000	P. Samuel Pegram, Jr., M.D. '70
2000	Henry Miller, M.D. '54
2001	C. Douglas Maynard, M.D. '59
2002	Brenda Latham-Sadler, M.D. '82

(continued from Distinguished Achievement Award)

1995	Spencer P. Thornton, MD '54
1996	Wilbur S. Avant, Jr., MD '67
1996	David Lowell Heymann, MD '70
1997	James S. Forrester, Sr., MD '62
1997	Godfrey P. Oakley, MD '65
1998	David P. Huston, MD '73
1999	William H. Admirand, MD '60
1999	Carolyn R. Ferree, MD '70
2000	George C. Barrett, M.D. '52
2000	H. Worth Boyce, Jr., M.D. '55
2001	Willliam N.P. Herbert, M.D. '72
2002	S. Scott Obenshain, M.D. '62

DISTINGUISHED SERVICE AWARD

1977	Thomas M. Holder, MD '52
1978	D. E. Ward, Jr., MD '45
1979	Manson Meads, MD
1981	A. C. Carpenter, MD
1982	John F. Watlington, Jr.
1983	J. Ralph Scales, Ph.D.
1984	D. E. Ward, Jr., MD '45
1984	Albert L. Butler
1985	Richard Janeway, MD, FHO
1986	Thomas H. Davis
1986	Jean Bailey Brooks, MD '44
1987	Claude A. McNeill, MD '43
1988	J. Paul Sticht
1989	Herbert Brenner
1990	Dixie Lee Boney Soo, MD '59
1991	M. Frank Sohmer, MD '52
1991	Richard D. Snyder, MD '58
1992	Louis deSchweinitz Shaffner, MD, FHO
1993	Kyle A. Young, MD '69
1993	Class of 1958

Distinguished Alumni Lecturers

1970

Dr. Jerry K. Aikawa, professor of medicine, University of Colorado School of Medicine, Denver (BG '45)

Col. H. Worth Boyce Jr., chief of the gastronterology service, Walter Reed Hospital, Washington, D. C. (BG '55)

Dr. Nancy C. Kester, associate professor of rehabilitation medicine, New York University School of Medicine, New York City (BG '55)

Dr. Robert L. Vann, associate medical development director, E. R. Squibb and Sons, Inc., Bristol, Tenn. (BG '45)

1971

Dr. Richard Burack, internist in North Conway, N.H. (BG '51)

Dr. S. Richardson Hill, vice president for health affairs, University of Alabama Medical Center, Birmingham (BG '46)

Dr. John A. Oates, professor of medicine and director of the Division of Clinical Pharmacology, Vanderbilt University School of Medicine (BG '56)

1972

Dr. Campbell W. McMillan, professor of pediatrics, University of North Carolina School of Medicine (BG '52)

Dr. Joyce H. Reynolds, on the emergency room staff, Forsyth Memorial Hospital (BG '52)

Dr. Oscar L. Sapp III, professor of medicine and associate dean for continuing education, UNC School of Medicine (BG '47)

1973

Dr. William B. Hunt, Jr., professor of medicine, University of Virginia School of Medicine, Charlottesville, Va., (BG '53)

Dr. Edwin H. Martinat, clinical associate professor of orthopedic surgery, Bowman Gray School of Medicine of Wake Forest University (BG '48)

Dr. James C. Hunt, associate director for clinical education programs, division of education, Mayo Foundation, Rochester, Minn. (BG '53)

1974

Dr. Donald M. Hayes, professor and chairman, department of community medicine, associate professor of medicine, Bowman Gray School of Medicine (BG '54)

Dr. James L. Quinn III, director of nuclear medicine, Northwestern Memorial Hospital, Chicago, IL (BG '59)

Dr. C. Glenn Sawyer, professor of medicine, Bowman Gray School of Medicine (BG '44)

1975

Dr. F. Murray Carroll, general practitioner, Chadbourn, North Carolina (BG '55)

Dr. Frederick Glass, assistant professor of surgery, acting head, section on emergency medical services, Bowman Gray School of Medicine, (BG '50)

Dr. J. Kiffin Penry, chief, applied neurologic research branch, collaborative an Field research, National Institute of Neurological and Communicative Disorders and Stroke, Bethesda, Maryland (BG '55)

Dr. Douglas H. Sandberg, professor of pediatrics and co-director, Clinical Research Center, University of Miami, Miami, Florida (BG '55)

1976

Dr. W. Eugene Cornatzer, professor and chairman, Department of Biochemistry, Director, Ireland Research Laboratory, University of North Dakota School of Medicine, Grand Forks, North Dakota (BG '51)

Dr. Marcus M. Gulley, associate professor of psychiatry, Bowman Gray School of Medicine (BG '51)

Dr. William Hudson, professor and chief, Division of Otolaryngology, Duke University Medical Center, Durham, North Carolina (BG '51)

Dr. William T. McLean, associate professor of neurology and pediatrics, Bowman Gray School of Medicine (BG '51)

1977

Dr. Thomas M. Holder, pediatric surgeon, clinical professor of surgery, University of Missouri at Kansas City, Missouri (BG '52)

Dr. M. Frank Sohmer, Jr., practitioner in gastroenterology and endoscopy. Clinical assistant professor of medicine, Bowman Gray School of Medicine (BG '52)

Dr. Wilbur C. Thomas, Pathologist, Meadville, Pennsylvania, assistant professor of pathology, 1943-47, Bowman Gray School of Medicine, associate professor Temple University, '47-51, associate professor, UCLA, '51-55 (BG-'37)

1978

Dr. Paul P. Griffin, professor and chairman of the Department of Orthopedics and Rehabilitation at Vanderbilt University Medical Center (BG '53)

Dr. William B. Herring, associate professor of medicine and chief of the University of North Carolina teaching programs at Moses H. Cone Memorial Hospital, Greensboro, North Carolina (BG '53)

Dr. Julian F. Keith, professor and chairman of the Department of Family and Community Medicine at Bowman Gray, Winston-Salem, North Carolina (BG '53)

1979

Dr. Donald M. Hayes, professor and chairman of the Department of Community Medicine at the University of Texas Health Science Center at Houston, Texas, recently joined Burlington Industries as medical director (BG '54).

Dr. Henry S. Miller, Jr., professor of medicine (cardiology) at Bowman Gray School of Medicine, Winston-Salem, North Carolina (BG '54)

1980

Dr. Joseph E. Whitley, professor and chairman of the Department of Radiology at the Unviersity of Marlayn School of Medicine (BG '55)

Dr. Richard B. Patterson, professor of pediatrics; (BG '55)

Dr. J. Kiffin Penry, professor of neurology and associate dean for neuroscience development (BG '55)

1981

Dr. David M. Drylie, professor and chief of the Division of Urology at the University of Florida College of Medicine; (BG-'56)

Dr. John H. Edmonds, professor of medicine (cardiology) at Bowman Gray (BG '56)

Dr. John S. Kaufmann, associate professor of medicine and pharmacology at Bowman Gray (BG '56)

1982

Dr. Mary Jo Carter, professor medicine at the Medical College of Georgia (BG '57)

Dr. W. Ray Cowan, director of the Armed Forces Institute of Pathology in Washington, D. C. (BG '57)

Dr. Nancy O. Whitley, professor of diagnostic radiology at the University of Maryland School of Medicine (BG '57)

1983

Dr. Glen E. Garrison, professor of medicine and family practice and director of continuing education at the Medical College of Georgia (BG '58)

Dr. Robert C. McKone, associate professor of pediatrics at Bowman Gray

Dr. Thomas J. Walsh, professor of ophthalmology and neurology at Yale University School of Medicine (BG '58)

1984

Dr. John D. Hines, professor of medicine at Case Western Reserve University School of Medicine (BG '59)

Dr. C. Douglas Maynard, professor and chairman of the Department of Radiology at Bowman Gray (BG '59)

1985

Dr. Lewis W. Thompson of City of Faith Medical and Research Center in Tulsa, Oklahoma (BG '60)

Dr. Robert E. Jones, associate professor of dermatology at the University of Alabama School of Medicine in Birmingham (BG '60)

Dr. Curtis L. Bakken, director of the Mayo Medical Laboratories in Rochester, Minnesota (BG '60)

Dr. Douglass F. Adams, professor of radiology and director of nuclear magnetic resonance at Harvard Medical School in Boston (BG '60)

Dr. Timothy C. Pennell, professor of surgery and director of the Office of International Health Affairs at Bowman Gray (BG '60)

1986

Dr. John M. Tew Jr., professor and chairman of the Department of Neurosurgery at the University of Cincinnati Medical Center (BG '61)

Dr. Charles E. McCall, professor of medicine and microbiology and head of the Section of Infectious Diseases at Bowman Gray (BG '61)

1987

Dr. John W. Reed, associate professor of surgery (ophthalmology) (BG '62)

Dr. Lloyd H. Harrison, professor of surgery (urology) (BG '62)

Dr. M. Robert Cooper, professor of medicine (hematology/oncology) (BG '62)

Dr. Ralph deS. Siewers, associate professor surgery at the University of Pittsburgh School of Medicine (BG '62)

Dr. William T. Carpenter, Jr., professor of psychiatry at the Maryland Psychiatric Research Center (BG '62)

Dr. John M. Driscoll, Jr., professor of clinical pediatrics at the Babies Hospital/Presbyterian Hospital of Columbia University College of physicians and Surgeons (BG '62)

Dr. S. Scott Obenshain, associate dean for undergraduate medical education at the University of New Mexico School of Medicine (BG '62)

1988

Dr. H. Garrett Adams, associate professor of pediatrics and director of the infectious disease section at the University of Louisville School of Medicine (BG '63)

Dr. Malcolm T. Foster, professor of medicine at the University of Florida College of Medicine (BG '63)

Dr. James L. Hughes, professor of orthopedic surgery at the University of Mississipi School of Medicine (BG '63)

Dr. Richard H. McShane of St. Barnabas Medical Center in Livingston, NJ (BG '63)

Dr. Richard B. Odom, professor of dermatology at the Medical Center of the University of California (BG '63)

1990

Dr. J. Bruce Smith, professor of medicine, microbiology and immunology at Jefferson Medical College in Philadelphia (BG '65)

Dr. Godfrey P. Oakley, Jr., director of the Division of Birth Defects and Developmental Disabilities at the Centers for Disease Control in Atlanta (BG '65)

Dr. Duke B. Weeks, professor of anesthesia at Bowman Gray and Brogdon. (BG '65)

1991

Dr. John M. Tew, Jr., professor and chairman of the Department of Neurosurgery at The University of Cincinnati College of Medicine (BG '61)

Dr. Franklin C. Wagner, Jr., professor and chairman of the Department of Neurological Surgery at the University of California, Davis, School of Medicine (BG '66)

Alpha Omega Alpha BETA CHAPTER OF NORTH CAROLINA

Alpha Omega Alpha (AOA) national honor medical society. No more than one-sixth of the graduating class can be elected to AOA.

Elected in 1950 – 1951 Graduates

Aikawa, Jerry K.
Avera, John W.
Aycock, James B.
Bethea, William T.
Brenton, Harold L.
Brunt, Manly Y.
Early, I. Gordon
Eisenberg, Seymour
Glenn, Leland K.
Hamrick, Ladd W.
Harris, Carlton M.
Hays, Glenn B.
Hill, S. Richardson
Horn, Paul L.
Jones, Warren H.
Kay, Charlotte R.
McClure, Claude Jr.
Miller, Ronald E.
Nance, John W.
Pittman, Hal W.
Pope, James K.
Sawyer, C. Glenn
Shingleton, William
Smith, Loy C.
Spurling, Carrol L.
Sweel, Alexander
Vann, Robert L.
Will, Thomas A.

Students

Burack, Richard
Cornatzer, William E.
Freeman, David
Gantt, Clarence Leroy
Groat, Richard Arnold
Gulley, Marcus M.
Gwynn, Thomas Lea
Huntley, Robert Ross
Jemison, Howard Allan
Johnson, Livingston
Joyner, John Thomas
Miller, Horace W.
Mills, Randolph Dennis

Elected in 1951 - 1952

Bass, Shelton T.
Byrum, Graham V.
Carpenter, Harry M.
Hahn, Dorothy A.
Ledbetter, John W.
Reynolds, Joyce H.
Sacrinty, Nicholas W.
Schultz, Everett H. Jr.
Simmons, James Q. III
Team, Robert A.

Elected in 1952 - 1953

Holleman, Ivan L. Jr.
Keith, Julian F.
Lanier, John T.
McCullum, Donald E.
McCuen, William G.
McLeod, John A. Jr.

Peacock, Avon J. Jr.
Snider, Bobby E.
Strickland, William H. Jr.

Elected in 1953 - 1954

Bates, Harold B.
Boyette, Edward L.
Crouch, Robert P.
Massey, Thomas N.
Morris, John A.
Pool, Robert S.
Schiess, Robert J. Jr.
Wood, Donald O.

Elected in 1954 - 1955

Adcock, Lester
Covell, W.A.
Crowder, Marietta
Kester, Nancy C.
Penry, J. Kiffin
Taylor, John R.
Whitley, Joseph E.
Wood, Donald O.
Underdal, Robert G.
Webster, Paul D. III

Elected in 1955 - 1956

Foster, Bob M.
Fowler, William
Hill, Arthur T.
Kaufmann, John S.
Sellers, Philip A.
Stevens, Ed L.
Stuart, Hal M.

Elected in 1956-1957

Hartzog, Donald C. Jr.
Linder, William John
Maercks, Ralph Owen
Moose, Lathan Thomas
Parker, Earl Wingate
Titmarsh, John Bailey
Watts, Lester Earl
York, Lowell Thomas

Elected in 1957 - 1958

Blackburn, John Thomas
Bronsky, Edwin Ansell
Fein, Arthur Leonard
Freidman, Stanley David
Jensen, Clayton Edward
Rish, Berkley Lamont
Rogers, John William
Soo, Dixie Boney
Weaver, George K.

Elected in 1958 - 1959

Boyette, Gray T.
Hines, John D.
Hoyme, James G.
Jones, Robert E. Jr.
Kitchen, Thomas W. Jr.
Mann, Robert F.
Myers, Fay K.
Quinn, James L. III

Elected in 1959 - 1960

Adams, Douglass Franklin
Admirand, William H.
Bakken, Curtis Leroy
Barber, George Curtis
Copeland, Gary Benjamin
Gatling, Hortense Bee
McCall, Charles Emory
Spencer, William Joseph
Tew, John McLelland Jr.

Elected in 1960 - 1961

Biggers, William H.
Buie, Thomas E. Jr.
Cooper, Miles R.
Engstrom, Lincoln L.
Foster, Jack E.
Graham, Gloria F.
Hlavinka, Delbert J.
Lavender, Dick R.
Wilfert, James N.

Elected in 1961 - 1962

Adams, Richard Wesley
Feezor, Charles Noel Jr.
Godwin, Herman Allen Jr.
Lefler, Wade Hampton Jr.
Pulliam, Robert Parker
Siewers, Christiane Maria Frederike
Siewers, Ralph deSchweinitz

Elected in 1962-1963

Burleson, Richard Lee
Carter, Robert Wilson
Cohen, Stephen Gordon
Collins, Nancy Marie
Krikorian, John Harry
Lane, Frederick Carl
Lindesmith, Larry Alan
Moore, Holland Victor
Swanson, Marjorie Angela

Elected in 1963 - 1964

Chapman, Anthony Jay
Curl, Charles Wayne
Gaines, Edmund Pendleton
Hedger, Robert Willis
Johnson, Louise Craig
McCullough, David LeGarde
Mattucci, Kenneth Francis
Poole, Gordon Joseph

Elected in 1964 - 1965

Blackburn, Thomas R.
Bolt, W. Michael
Dacus, Robert M.
Fagen, Sheldon G.
Oakley, Godfrey P. Jr.
Puckett, Charles L.
Thorpe, Darrell P.

Elected in 1965 - 1966

Adcock, Eugene W. III
Allen, Elmo L.
Goode, David J.

Hamrick, John C. Jr.
McAlhany, Joseph C. Jr.
Picklesimer, Fred L.
Severy, Philip R.
Yarbrough, John W.

Elected in 1966 - 1967

Ball, Marshall R.
Bisecker, James L.
Martin, Gerry D.
Schiller, Herbert M.
Self, James L.
Smithson, W. Anthony
Thompson, John A. Jr.
Tullock, E. Franklin Jr.
Wallace, Wilson K.

Elected in 1967 - 1968

Hamill, Robert W.
Herring, R. McPhail
LeGrand, Robert H.
McGuirt, William F.
Phillips, John A.
Smith, Samuel N.
Speck, William T.
Taylor, Julian R.

Elected in 1968 - 1969

Bean, S. Charles
Buchanan, Robert A.
Harris, Jimmy G.
King, Charles E. Jr.
McAlister, James A. Jr.
Pridgen, Durward B.
Resnick, Martin I.
Woods, Monty
Young, Kyle A.

Elected in 1969 - 1970

Alexander, Charles F. III
Burch, Warner M. Jr.
Casey, William J.
Hensley, Michael J.
Heymann, David L.
Pegram, P. Samuel Jr.
Purnell, W. David
Reddick, Lovett P.
Shelly, Donald W.

Elected in 1970 - 1971

Baird, Frances G.
Davis, Ben K.
Fleming, Duard F. Jr.
Godehn, D. John Jr.
Hensen, Keith S.
Hunt, Thomas H.
Karotkin, Edward H.
Latham, Andrew W.
Whisnant, Joseph D.

Elected in 1971 - 1972

Bloom, John D.
Gallup, Kenneth R. Jr.
Hardy, John G.
Hoyle, James C. Jr.

Knott, Lawrence H. Jr.
McDonald, Bruce B.
McLeskey, Charles H.
Poole, Terry W.
Reynolds, R. Neal
Winstead, Laura L.

Elected in 1972 - 1973

Ashburn, Philip E.
Blackwell, David E.
Burgess, Grace S.
Butler, Robert H.
Kosinski, Edward J.
Marks, Eric S.
Oliver, David C.
Paschal, George W. III
Plonk, George W. Jr.
Rouse, John L. III
Simpson, John L.
Vidinghoff, Robert P.

Elected in 1973 - 1974

Dobner, Joseph J.
Haponik, Edward F.
Kelly, John S.
Lambeth, William R.
Marx, Richard S.
Miller, Joel B.
Rogers, James D.
Scruggs, Michael C.
Shoaf, Edwin H. Jr.
Sink, James D.
Strohecker, James S.
Walley, Bruce D.

Elected in 1974 - 1975

Alsbrook, Everett H. Jr.
Anderson, Theodore S. Jr.
Atkinson, James B.
Berg, Alan M.
Boyette, Douglas R.
Burnette, J. P.
Ginn, Thomas M.
Gulledge, Sidney L. III
O'Neill, Michael R.
Spees, Lynn B.
Spurr, Charles L. Jr.
Tinga, John H.
Wexler, Donald
Woodall, Hal B.

Elected in 1975 - 1976

Bagwell, Charles E.
Baldwin, Phillip E.
Beyer, Fred C.
Broughton, Robert A.
Bryant, James E.
Cline, Wayne A.
Edwards, Joel L.
Harlan, Joseph E. Jr.
Holland, Walter B.
Kasperik, Donald J.
Kelly, Richard J.
Lupton, George P.
Rose, Paula G.
Williamson, Roberta A.

Elected in 1976 - 1977

Beazley, Luther A. III
Black, Richard A.
Bradley, Joel F. Jr.
Detlefs, Richard L.
Dolson, Ellen M.
Gates, Robert H.
Krowchuk, Daniel P.
Levinson, Mark M.
McKay, Charles E. III
Meredith, J. Mark J. III
Mustol, John S.
Myers, Mark S.
Ogburn, Nicholas L.
Paschold, Eugene H.
Peterson, Robert C.
Snyder, Bruce A.
Vogler, James B. III

Elected in 1977 - 1978

Ash, Nancy L.
Baker, James D. III
Beatty, Lee A.
Butterfield, Jack D.
Lentz, Samuel S.
Linton, Frances J.
Lowery, Gayla S.
Sachs, Stephen S.
Sievers, Richard E.
Tennant, Stanley N.
Wallenhaupt, Stephen L.

Elected in 1978 - 1979

Baker, Alfred L.
Berger, Jack L.
Caldwell, David C.
Cloninger, Karen G.
Clontz, Ted H.
Colavita, Paul G.
Hawks, Al N. Jr.
Honeycutt, Danny M.
Knauer, William J.
Matthews, Brian L.
Pugh, Walter L.
Rahm, Robin L.
Robinson, Edward N.
Smith, Vernon C.
Stetler, Robert H.
Tilley, William S.
Troxell, Marcus L.

Elected in 1979 - 1980

Allen, Benjamin G.
Appler, Mark L.
Hix, Mark T.
Howe, Harold R. Jr.
Liverman, Joseph T. Jr.
Matsumoto, Alan H.
Mayron, Raymond
McComb, John S.
Parrish, Edward J.
Peterman, Angela R.
Salberg, Jeffrey P.
Sowers, John C.
Wilson, Marguerite T.
Van Zandt, Keith B.

Volosin, Kent J.
Warren, Richard C.

Elected in 1980 - 1981

Brooks, C. Michael
Davis, Owen K.
Edgerton, T. Arthur
Holland, N. Wilson Jr.
Kent, Brian D.
Lineberger, Adrian S.
Matthews, Karen B.
McAlpine, Robert G. Jr.
Nave, L. David Jr.
Pate, Marion B. III
Penley, W. Charles
Sawada, Kathleen Y.
Schreiber, David P.
Smith, Thomas C.
West, Laura P.
Williams, C. David

Elected in 1981 - 1982

Annand, David W.
Culp, Pamela J.
Gotchel, Mark P.
Hiatt, J. Donald Jr.
Jacobs, William A.
Kutler, Marc S.
Labs, J. Daniel
Mangum, Michael D.
Mills, Michael K.
Murphy, John B. Jr.
Reid, Richard H.
Rich, Charles B.
Rosner, Diane R.
Updike, Sarah M.
Wall, Thomas C.
Wehbie, Charles B.
Wiggins, Thomas B.
Williams, Nancy L.

Elected in 1982 - 1983

Connolly, Brian M.
Greven, Craig M.
Harr, Charles D.
Herrick, Timothy W.
Hodnett, Cynthia R.
Huntsman, W. Thomas
Jones, Charles M. III
Kammire, Gordon C.
Krahnert, John F. Jr.
Kruger, Karolyn S.
Maynard, C. Douglas, M.D.
Faculty
Mills, Melissa J.
Rhyne, Janelle A.
Tanner, S. Bobo IV
Tyson, Archie A. Jr.
White, Kenneth S.
Young, William F. Jr.

Elected in 1983 - 1984

Cermak, Jill P.
Feehs, Kimberly D.
Fernandez, Gonzalo G.
Hartsell, F. Wright

Jeffries, Deborah O.
McMaster, Mary L.
Moore, Robert A. III
Nelson, Leonard D. Jr.
Raines, Karen H.
Smith, Douglas K.
Snyder, H. Dennis III
Trahey, Thomas F.
White, Kevin M.
Widman, Stephen C.
Willard, Ellen M.
Williford, Susan K.

Elected in 1984 - 1985

Burger, Charles D.
Collins, R. Andrew
Copeland, Carol E.
Dale, Wheeler J.
Flynn, Charles L.
Fowler, Fred C.
Fowler, Wyatt C.
Freimanis, Rita I.
Gee, Michael L.
Gerard, Craig J.
Hornbeck, Robert G.
Pence, Carla R.
Walker, G. Kirk
Wardell, Donald M. III
Wells, Steven R.

Elected in 1985 - 1986

Amick, Martin
Aronson, Richard
Daltner, Carl
Davis, John
Fowler, Fred
Gibson, Brian
Hammet, Chris
Hott, Kim
Iles, Donna
Kammire, Leslie
Overbey, Warren
Owen, William
Purgason, Polly
Samuels, Larry
Schafer, Gary
Shafran, Kerry
Walsh, Frank

Elected in 1986 - 1987

Barton, John H. Jr.
Boyette, Frances
Chandler, Howard C. Jr.
Collins, Diana B.
Daddabbo, Joseph G.
Dresser, Lee P.
Ellington, Charles P. III
Heavner, Teresa A.
Kontis, Theda C.
Liebscher, Gregory J.
McCain, Brenda L.
Sandberg, Eric T.
South, Stephen A.
Spivey, David E. Jr.
Vollger, Helmuth F.
Wilson, Jesse R.

Elected in 1987 - 1988

Baumgarner, Laurie S.
Caldwell, George L. Jr.
Claussen, Gwendolyn C.
Cole, Roger D.
Dimmette, Pattie J.
Dugger, Karen K.
Eaton, Jeffrey G.
Ferrall, Robert J.
Gower, Verlia C.
Hill, Thomas R.
Kramer, Jane K.
LaMay, Edward N.
Lord, Richard W. Jr.
Mack, Yvonne
Rathmell, James P.
Ruch, David S.
Verschuyl, Evert J.

Elected in 1988 - 1989

Brody, Jeffrey Arnold
Crum, Amy Elizabeth
Darnell, Linda Ruth
Epstein, Susan Elise
Golding, Eugene Marion Jr.
Ireland, Patrick David
Johnson, Allen McKenzie
Kouri, David Lawrence
Kuhr, Julie Francis
Lodge, Jeffrey
Riggin, Jasper Simmons III
Smith, Yolanda Regina
Standish, Myles Patrick
Stephenson, Anne Elizabeth
Waddell, Brad Edward
Wray, Anna Hopeman

Elected in 1989 - 1990

Alphin, Robert Stancil
Bandarenko, Nickolas III
Brady, Don Irvin
Cintron, Ruben
DiRocca, Judith Geralyn
Fuller, Stanley Brian
Key, Steven Paul
Lenhard, Julie Marie
Moose, Beverly Dawn
Myers, Wendell Stephen
Robaczewski, David Lee
Snyder, Lisa Beth
Stroud, Larry Ashley
Thomas, Christopher Crim
Whitaker, Robert Norton Jr.

Elected in 1990 - 1991

Atteberry, Linda Rose
Carty, Calphor Stanford
Chang, Edward Jinki
Chiu, Arva Yahua
Cotton, Christopher Douglas
Dickens, Mahlon Alan
Gallerani, Peter Mark
Gibson, Susan Holland
Kellam, Lori Goco
Khosla, Siddarth Mitter
Marshall, Harvey Edwin III

Orville, Stephen Wyatt
Paul, Amy Foster
Smith, Michael Scott
Steinberg, Martin Irwin
Stonehouse, Stephen Edward
Wilmoth, Gregory Jennings

Elected in 1991 - 1992

Berman, Lisa Anne
Bower, William Alfred
Coric, Domagoj
Eakins, Darrin Franklin
Gorsuch, Lisa Ann
Greelish, James Patrick
Jones, Charles Wade
Kreiter, Shelley Rae
Lewis, Kristin Helga
Mathews, Raymond M.
Modest, Vicki Ellen
Napper, Clay Hughes Jr.
Ramsey, Jenifer Ann
Rupard, Leslie Lynn
Stennette, Denise Suzanne
Wilson, Charles Jerome

Elected in 1992 - 1993

Abernethy, William B. III
Ardans, Tamara Marie
Castellion, Deena Manon
Connelley, Christopher Scott
Crook, Mary Elizabeth
Davis, Daniel Edwin
Eskew, Lawrence Andrew
Geyer, Anne Huggins
Hilowitz, Deborah Eve
Komada, Michael Rudolph
Miller, Preston Roy III
Nichols, George Louis Jr.
Noone, Tara Creedon
Quick, Rhonda Carol
Quistgaard, Susanne Ulrich
Scacheri, Robert Quinto
Steffee, Craig Harold
Van Hoy, Barbara Elizabeth

Elected in 1993 - 1994

Bowling, Jack W.
Brock, Margaret F.
Brodish, Brian N.
Clapp, Christopher R.
Collins, Ingeborg C.
Del Savio, Beth C.
Foster, M. Shane
Johnson, J. Theodore
Kincaid, Edward H.
Rogers, M. Sean
Schiller, Anne B.
Smith, Timothy E.
Taws, Kathy A.
Vann, Robin R.
Williams, Julie A.

Elected in 1994 - 1995

Anderson, Curtis Austin
Bohan, Michael Nolan
Burroughs, Arthur Andersen

Clark, Joseph Madison II
Holroyd, John Bailie
Jones, David Scott
Loehr, Steve Peter
McCain, Trent Winslow
McNeil, Cheryl Lynn
Mendiratta, Anil
Neville, Michael James
Ott, Susan J.
Oursler, Ralph Everett III
Peterman, Scott H.
Poehling, Katherine Anne
Reulbach, Todd Russell
Rozzelle, Curtis J.
Shappley, Nora Catherine
Winter, Jerald L.
Abramson, Jon S., M.D.,
  Faculty
Elster, Allen, M.D.,
  Faculty
Ely, Kim, M.D.,
  House Officer
Hines, Mike, M.D.,
  House Officer
Lauve, Lucie, M.D.,
  House Officer

Elected in 1995 - 1996

Averill, Kevin Jay
Boord, Jeffrey Barton
Campbell, Kevin Ray
Corley, Bonnie Sierra
Foote, John Derrell
George, Christopher Michael
Guerrero, John Miguel
Klein, Bert Jack
Moody, Laurel Hutchison
Poate, Timothy James
Purser, Constance Beth
Rusyniak, Daniel Edward
Talley, Rebecca Ann
Taylor, Priscilla Renee
Warren, Deborah Parry
Webb, Leslie Anne
Zopp, Amanda Jane
Baker, Albert M., M.D.,
  House Officer
Seaton, Anthony, M.D.,
  House Officer
Smith, John Matthew, M.D.,
  House Officer
Adams, Patricia L., M.D.,
  Faculty
Ober, K. Patrick, M.D.,
  Faculty

Elected in 1996 - 1997

Albright, Mark Phillip
Barker, Timothy Andrew
DeMars, Carl Sinai
Elnicky, Carol Jean
Ferriss, David Michael
Gessner, Martin Thomas
Gorman, Richard Forbes
Jones, Timothy Royal
Jordan, Mark Kenneth

Kim, Eugene Jacob
McDonald, John Matthew
Melisko, Michelle Elizabeth
Noud, Michael John
Olsen, Amy
Ott, Michael Clifford
Price, Kenneth Owen
Ray, Richard Mark
Stone, Jeffrey Davis
Teal, Lara Jean
Loughlin, Christopher James, M.D.
  House Officer
White, Benjamin T., M.D.,
  House Officer
Thompson, James N., M.D.
  Faculty

Elected in 1997 - 1998

Aldridge, Julian McClees
Berghausen, Elizabeth Katherin
Dittrich, Lee Baxter
Epps, Lori Birana
Fahey, Sean Michael
Howe, David Jefferson
Hughes, Michael Gerald
Page, Mary Elizabeth
Pardini, Ricci Stefan
Perini, Mark Andrew
Pruden, Charles Howell
Sandhu, Haspreet Singh
Satterfield, William Harper
Smith, Edward Shiang-Lin
Stull, Dennis Francis
Sumner, Brian
Xie, Sean Xiaorong
Dunagan, Donnie, M.D.
  House Officer
Cruz, Julia, M.D.
  Faculty
Reifler, Burton, M.D.
  Faculty

Elected in 1998 - 1999

Bennett-Cain, Andrea
Brady, Paul
Buckley, Kevin
Bullard, Carlin
Chen, Randolph
Clyne, Stephen
Collins, Andrew
Cooper, Jennifer
Dillmon, Melissa Stuart
Hanna, Christine
Hughes, Michael
Marlowe-Rogers, Heidi
Michener, Michael
Nance, Christopher
Niblack, Brett
Redmon, Eric
Russell, Hyde
Scherer, Kerri
Schweickert, William
Sheppert, Andrew
Wares, Jennifer
Agner, Christopher, M.D.
  Community-based Faculty

Cannon, Mark, M.D.
  House Officer
Das, Saurabh, M.D.
  House Officer
Lee, Linda, M.D.
  House Officer
Namen, Andrew, M.D.
  House Officer
Meredith, Wayne, M.D.
  Alumni
Miller, Henry, M.D.
  Alumni
Roufail, Walter, M.D.
  Faculty
Troost, Todd, M.D.
  Faculty

Elected in 1999 - 2000

Bashinsky, Alice
Burns, Cynthia
Donlevy, Elisabeth
Frino, John
Ginn, Adam
Gregory, Alexia
Hockey, Karen
Jones, Lyell
Lesslie, Gretel
Martin, David
Miller, Suzanne
Neale, Christine
Powers, Heather
Schneider, Tim
Simmons, Jeff
Swayne, David
Turner, Elizabeth
Urioste, Alex
Nifong, Ted, M.D.
  House Officer
Johnson, Jeri, M.D.
  House Officer
McElderry, Hugh, M.D.
  House Officer
Weaver, Jim, M.D.
  House Officer
Dolinski, Sylvia, M.D.
  Faculty
Pryor, Elizabeth, M.D.
  Faculty

Elected in 2000 - 2001

Bates, Dwight David
Buroker, Jane Wainscott
Clark, Julie Christine
Grosvenor, Alexandra
  Rowland
Horton, Janet Knight
Jacks, Karen Elizabeth
Martin, Robert Shayn
Mazie, Karen Barclay
Millender, Laura Ellen
Peral, Lindsay Seawright
Phan, Melanie Ngochan
Powers, Brent Michael
Quartermain, Michael David
Rees, Catherine Jane
Smith, Jennifer Green

Streck, Maria Rudisill
Underhill, Hunter Reeve
West, Thomas Graham
Wiley, Virginia Carolyn
Jones, Brandy
  House Officer
Lepak, Jason
  House Officer
Kirkman, Paul
  Alumni
Latham-Sadler, Brenda
  Alumni
MacGregor, Drew
  Faculty
Shaw, Ed
  Faculty

Elected in 2001 - 2002

Anderson, Steven
Boyd, Michael
Cartwright, Michael
Cartwright, Sarah
Eagleson, Elizabeth
Faler, Byron
Funk, Wendy
Inman, Lucas
Krawitz, Seth
Long, Amy
Moore, Phillip
Ramsey, Ashley
Roberts, Christine
Rubin, Diana
Shahine, Lora
Thompson, Christine
Toenjes, Steve
Preli, Bob, M.D.
  House Staff
Priest, David, M.D.
  House Staff
Jackson, David, M.D.
  Alumni
Rice, Billy, M.D.
  Alumni
Lawless, Michael, M.D.
  Faculty

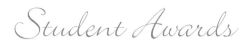

Student Awards

DR. MARTIN AND SANDRA CASTLEBAUM AWARD FOR EXCELLENCE IN INTERNAL MEDICINE

(formerly the Tinsley Harrison Internal Medicine Award)
— Presented to the graduating senior, selected by the Department of Internal Medicine, who demonstrates outstanding abilities and exceptional potential in the field of internal medicine

1990	Larry Ashley Stroud
1991	Harvey Edwin Marshall III
1992	William Alfred Bower
1993	Daniel Edwin Davis
	Michael Rudolph Komada
1994	Phillip Ray Morrow
1995	John Holroyd
1996	Constance B. Purser
1997	Richard F. Gorman
1998	Mark Andrew Perini
	Melissa Mazzini Zorn
1999	Randolph Alan Chen
2000	Karen Joy Hockey
	Elizabeth Edwards Turner
2001	Brent Michael Powers
2002	Elizabeth Ann Eagleson

CHARLES BRIAN CLARK MEMORIAL AWARD

— Given by the senior medical students in memory of former student Charles B. Clark to someone who has provided outstanding service to the class

1991	June G. May
1992	Michael R. Lawless
1993	Brenda Befus
1994	Cam Enarson
1995	Lynn Snyder
1996	Robert Petrilli
1997	Elizabeth Sherertz
1998	Edward Haponik
1999	Lynn Snyder
2000	K. Patrick Ober
2001	Melissa L. Stevens
2002	Kevin Brewer

C.B. DEANE MEMORIAL AWARD

— Presented to the student whose performance in clinical oncology has been most outstanding

1971	William Lee Ramseur Jr.
1972	Eric Charles Nelson
	Hugh Toland Stoddard Jr.
1973	J. Laurence Ransom
	Charles W. Scarantino
1974	Philip Eugene Ashburn
	David Samuel Stephens
1975	David Earl Davenport
1976	Fred C. Beyer
1977	Mary Marvin Johnson
	Mark E. Ellis
1978	Philip O. Katz
	Gayla S. Lowery
1979	Paul G. Colavita
	John J. Maloney III
1980	Edward J. Parrish
1981	David P. Schreiber
	Thomas C. Smith
1982	Michael D. Mangum
1983	Kathryn M. Greven
	Melissa J. Mills
1984	Robert A. Moore III
1985	Aaron V. Kaplan
1986	Robert E. Hersh
1987	Maury M. Rosenstein
1988	Alan B. Clark
1989	James J. Kinahan
1990	David Raben
1991	Lisa Allyn Boardman
1992	Clay Hughes Napper Jr.
1993	Stephanie Murphy Duggins
1994	Christopher A. Philippart
1995	John Holroyd
1996	Kevin Ray Campbell
	Philip Ashley Parser
1997	Mark A. Perini
1998	Samantha J. Pulliam
	Mark A. Perini
1999	Melissa Stuart Dillmon
2000	Evan Daniel Gross
2001	Janet Knight Horton
2002	Michael Allison Nichols

EXCELLENCE IN DERMATOLOGY AWARD

— Presented to the graduating student whose interaction with the faculty in the Department of Dermatology best exemplifies leadership, intellectual ability, achievement, and humanity

1992	John Stephen Wikle	1998	Edward S. Smith
1993	Victoria Bradford Mawn	1999	Carlin Nicole Bullard
1994	Beth Del Savio	2000	Reem Samir Utterback
1995	Ann Thomas Sutton	2001	Sarah La Truong
1996	Darryl S. Hodson	2002	Manisha Jashbhai Patel
1997	Susanna B. Bleyer		

FACULTY AWARD

— Given by the faculty to a graduating student who has demonstrated overall scholarship and character during four years of medical education

1960	Fay Knickerbocker Myers	1982	Owen K. Davis
1961	Charles Emory McCall	1983	Melissa J. Mills
1962	James Norris Wilfert	1984	Karolyn S. Kruger
1963	Herman Allen Godwin Jr.	1985	Gonzalo G. Fernandez
1964	Richard Lee Burleson	1986	William C. Owen
1965	Robert Mabry Dacus III	1987	Diana B. Collins
1966	Darrell Phelps Thorpe	1988	Jeffrey G. Eaton
1967	John Ward Yarbrough	1989	Eugene M. Golding Jr.
1968	James Leland Self	1990	Beverly Dawn Moose
1969	Rufus McPhail Herring Jr.	1991	Lori Goco Kellam
1970	William Joseph Casey	1992	William Alfred Bowen
1971	Edward Harvey Karotkin	1993	Preston Roy Miller and
1972	Deward Francis Fleming Jr.		Craig Harold Steffee
1973	Edward J. Kosinski	1994	Timothy Earl Smith
1974	Philip Eugene Ashburn	1995	Anil Mendiratta
1975	James David Sink	1996	Priscilla R. Taylor
1976	Alan M. Berg	1997	Kenneth O. Price
1977	Richard J. Kelly	1998	Lori B. Epps
1978	Eugene H. Paschold	1999	Heidi Cruz Marlowe-Rogers
1979	Jack D. Butterfield Jr.	2000	Elizabeth Edwards Turner
1980	Edward J. Parrish	2001	Alexandra Rowland Grosvenor
1981	John C. Sowers	2002	Lola Padgitt Kelly

I. MESCHAN RADIOLOGY MERIT AWARD

— Presented in honor of Isadore Meschan, M.D., renowned radiologist and chair of the Department of Radiology for 22 years (1955-1977), to a student who has performed outstanding research and demonstrated academic excellence in radiology

1995	Stephen P. Loehr	2000	William Tom Kuo
1998	John N. Campbell	2001	Elaine Grace Khatod
1999	Mark Davidson Hiatt	2002	Lance Edward Driskill

MATSUMAE AWARD

— Given to a senior medical student who has demonstrated compassion and interest in international understanding. President Shigeyoshi Matsumae of Tokai University in Japan and the Matsumae International Foundation presented the Matsumae trophy to the School of Medicine in September 1988 in recognition of the establishment of cooperative educational and research programs between Tokai University and our School of Medicine.

1989	Ziaollah Hashemi	1997	Sherri D. Campbell
1990	Monty Stephen Ledbetter		Suzanne E. Mitchell
1991	Josef Francis Schmid	1998	Jaspreet S. Singh
1992	Manisha Satish Ashar	1999	Julia Kirsten Roos
1993	Ulfur Thorbjorns Gudjonsson	2000	Alexander Joseph Davit
1994	Tatsuro Ogisu	2001	Anita Katherine King
1995	Shiva Jarrahi Kincaid	2002	Michael R. Savona
1996	James R. High		

MEDICAL ALUMNI ASSOCIATION EXCELLENCE AWARD

(Formerly called the Achievement Award)

— Presented to the member of the senior class who, as determined by ballot of classmates, best personifies the "ideal" doctor

1969	Julian Raleigh Taylor	1988	Jeffrey G. Eaton
1970	Paul Samuel Pegram Jr.		Richard W. Lord Jr.
1971	Edward Harvey Karotkin	1989	Richard J. Dobyns
1972	Leon Festus Woodruff Jr.	1990	John Franklin Davis
1973	Edward J. Kosinski	1991	Maria Sgambati
1974	Philip Eugene Ashburn	1992	Charles Wade Jones
1975	Edwin Huss Shoaf Jr.	1993	Mary Elizabeth Crook
1976	George P. Lupton		Lawrence Andrew Eskew
1977	James B. Vogler III	1994	Amy Barta Wall
1978	Eugene H. Paschold	1995	David Jones
1979	Jack E. Butterfield Jr.	1996	John D. Foote
1980	Ted H. Clontz	1997	Jeffrey D. Stone
1981	Mark T. Hix	1998	Keith Demond Gray
1982	Thomas C. Wall		Dennis Francis Stull
1983	Andrew S. Griffin	1999	Kevin Stuart Buckley
1984	Archie A. Tyson Jr.	2000	Lyell Keen Jones
1985	Wyatt C. Fowler	2001	Dwight David Bates
1986	Fred C. Fowler	2002	Michael Stephen Cartwright
1987	Daphne Bicket		

M. ROBERT COOPER SCHOLARSHIP AWARD

— Presented in honor of Dr. Cooper, longtime faculty member and esteemed oncologist, to a medical student who has performed pertinent research in the field of oncology

1983	Kay Lahon	1993	William McCall Brinkley
1984	Archie A. Tyson (Zan)	1994	Rodwige Jacques Desnoyers
1985	Michael J. C. McNamara	1995	Nancy L. Mooradian
1986	Leslie D. Kammire	1996	Suzanne E. Mitchell
1987	James P. Rathmell	1997	Michelle E. Melisko
1988	Gretchen G. Kimmick	1998	Jawan C. Ayer
1989	Douglas A. Fein	1999	Eric Thomas Mullen
1990	Beverly Dawn Moose	2000	Michael Alex Papagikos
1991	Maria Sgambati	2001	Ashley Ford Ramsey
1992	Lillian Hamilton Rinker	2002	Amret Elizabeth Thompson

OBSTETRICS AND GYNECOLOGY MERIT AWARD

— Presented by the faculty of the Department of Obstetrics and Gynecology to the student who exhibits the most outstanding academic and professional stature

1962	Robert Parker Pulliam	1983	Charles M. Jones III
1963	John Harry Krikorian	1984	Laura L. Williams
1964	Richard Lee Burleson	1985	William C. Rawls Jr.
1965	Robert Mabry Dacus III	1986	Warren M. Overbey
1966	David Nimmons Smith	1987	Charles P. Ellington III
1967	Earl Franklin Tulloch Jr.	1988	David A. Barkley
1968	William Frederick McGuirt	1989	Luther H. Eure Jr.
1969	James Allen McAlister Jr.	1990	George Craig Clinard
1970	Paul Samuel Pegram Jr.	1991	Fredrik Lars Jarskog
1971	Don Jennings Hall	1992	Lisa Ann Gorsuch
1972	Louis Weinstein	1993	Mary Elizabeth Crook
1973	Paul A. Holyfield	1994	Ingeborg Connelly Collins
1974	John Milton Roberts Jr.	1995	Craig M. Martin
1975	John Hinnes Tinga	1996	Bonnie S. Corley
1976	Stephen H. Cruikshank	1997	John M. McDonald
1977	James E. Ferguson II	1998	Andrew J. Lewis
1978	Marlene F. Kaniuk	1999	Kerri Renee Scherer
1979	Bruce L. Flamm	2000	Mary Suzanne Miller
1980	John S. McComb	2001	Jennifer Green Smith
1981	Vickie W. Lovin	2002	Lynda Gioia
1982	Owen K. Davis		

OUTSTANDING MEDICAL STUDENT IN PSYCHIATRY AWARD

— Presented by the Department of Psychiatry to the student whose performance in that field has been most commendable

1995	Susan Kostenko	2000	Eric Rashad Williams
1997	David E. Hardesty	2001	Karen Elizabeth Jacks
1998	Lori B. Epps	2002	Heston Channing LaMar
1999	Kala Cheryl Gray		

PEDIATRIC MERIT AWARD

— Given to the student selected by the pediatrics faculty as having the best all-around ability and interest in the care of children, not based on academic standing alone.

1957	Hervy Basil Kornegay
1958	Robert Clair McKone
1959	Arthur Leonard Fein
1960	H. Bee Gatling
1961	Thomas E. Buie
1962	Samuel Scott Obenshain
1963	John Harry Krikorian
1964	Wayne Carson Koontz
1965	Godfrey Porter Oakley, Jr.
1966	Roger Eugene Stevenson
1967	Stephen Jan Eberhard
1968	John Keenan Whisnant, Jr.
1969	John Atlas Phillips
1970	Charles Allen Bullaboy
1971	James Michael Rogers
1972	James Cranford Hoyle, Jr.
1973	William A. Fawcett IV
1974	Tracy Lee Trotter
1975	William Stevenson Browner
1976	Jon S. Abramson
1977	Daniel P. Krowchuk
1978	Susan R. Levy
1979	Julian F. Keith III
1980	Robert S. Ellison
1981	Adrian S. Lineberger
1982	Mary Ann Rozakis
1983	P. Charles Engstrom
1984	Karen H. Raines
1985	Kimberly D. Feehs
1986	Mary Beth Conway
1987	Anne E. Schreck
1988	Jeffrey G. Eaton
1989	Eugene M. Golding, Jr.
1990	Gian Paolo Bentivaglio
1991	Denise Pelham Tunstall
1992	Shelley Rae Kreiter
1993	Deborah Eve Hilowitz
1994	Christopher R. Clapp
1995	Catherine Shappley Mason
1996	Laurel H. Moody
1997	David C. Thomas
1998	Elizabeth K. Berghausen
1999	Pamela Kristina Cochran
2000	Gretel Lauren Lesslie
2001	Jane Wainscott Buroker
2002	Kevin Dennis Hill
	Amy Wilson Long

RICHARD L. BURT RESEARCH ACHIEVEMENT AWARD

— Presented to a medical student who has given a significant amount of time to research

1983	Charles M. Jones III		1993	William Borden Abernethy III
1985	William H. Kutteh		1994	Ramona Gelzer Bell
1986	Leslie D. Kammire		1995	Stephen P. Loehr
1987	Edward T. Chappell		1996	Patricia L. Turner
1988	Charles S. Clark		1997	Albert C. Lo
	James P. Rathmell		1998	Edward S. Smith
1989	Stephen F. Lewis		1999	Michael Gerald Hughes, Jr.
1990	David Lee Robaczewski		2001	Robert Shayn Martin
1992	Lemuel Broome Kirby		2002	Scott Allen Mayfield
	Stephen Ledbetter			

RICHARD T. MYERS SURGICAL MERIT AWARD

— Presented to the graduating student whose participation in surgery during medical school has been the most outstanding

1980	Harold R. Howe, Jr.
1981	T. Arthur Edgerton
1982	Richard J. Blinkhorn, Jr.
1983	Charles D. Harr
1984	R. Bradley Thomason III
1985	Ellen M. Willard
1986	Warren M. Overbey
1987	Brantley T. Jolly, Jr.
1988	Evert J. Verschuyl
1989	Jeffery S. Lodge
1990	David L. Robaczewski
1991	Linda Rose Atteberry
1992	Charles Wade Jones
1993	Preston Roy Miller
1994	Edward Hal Kincaid
1995	Curtis Anderson
1996	Kevin Jay Averill
1997	John C. Paschold
1998	William H. Satterfield
1999	Stephen Bernard Clyne
2000	Thomas Adam Ginn
2001	Robert Shayn Martin
2002	Michael Brian Boyd

ROBERT P. VIDINGHOFF MEMORIAL AWARD

— Presented to the graduating student who exhibits the greatest aptitude in and devotion to the field of family practice

1975	Samuel Baggett McLamb, Jr.
1976	Joel L. Edwards
1977	John B.R. Thomas
1978	Lee A. Beatty
1979	Jack D. Butterfield, Jr.
1980	Joseph T. Liverman, Jr.
1981	Laura Pinner West
1982	Joseph G. Taylor
1983	Steven M. Rachbach
1984	Perry L. Bartelt
1985	James P. Longe
1986	Nancy C. Winker
1987	David E. Spivey, Jr.
1988	Richard W. Lord, Jr.
1989	Richard J. Dobyns
1990	John Franklin Davis
1991	Robert Stark Adams
1992	Cynthia Jo Weisenauer
1993	Scott Howard Johnson
1994	Sara Lynn Neal
1995	Stephen G. Bissette
1996	Alisa C. Nance
1997	Lara J. Teal
1998	Alan D. Perry
1999	Heidi Cruz Marlowe-Rogers
2000	David William Swayne
2001	Lindsay Seawright Peral
2002	Sarah Lieber Cartwright

R. W. PRICHARD HISTORY OF MEDICINE AWARD

— Presented to a medical student who has written an outstanding paper on the history of medicine, the award is given in memory of Robert W. Prichard, M.D., faculty member for 44 years, distinguished chair of pathology, and respected medical historian.

1996	J. Brent Myers
	Kevin D. Lye
1997	Mark Davidson Hiatt
	Lara Junine Pons
1998	Samantha C. Timmons
	Jeffrey C. Constantine
	M. Suzanne Miller
1999	Kristine S. Vossler
	Charlie Ching Yang
2000	Rebecca Woods Daniel
	Munira Dabir Siddiqui
2001	Jeffrey Allen Vallee
	Geoffrey Alan Abell
2002	Samuel P. Jacks
	B. Rhys Lam

SAEM (SOCIETY FOR ACADEMIC EMERGENCY MEDICINE) MEDICAL STUDENT EXCELLENCE IN EMERGENCY MEDICINE AWARD

— Presented annually to the medical student in each U.S. medical school who best exemplifies the qualities of an excellent emergency physician, including excellent clinical, interpersonal, and manual skills, continuing professional development, and outstanding performance on emergency medical rotations

1992	William Shaun Gogarty
1993	Tamara Marie Ardans
1996	Kevin J. Averill
1997	Timothy H. Hurtzog
1998	J. Brent Myers
1999	Jennifer Bennett Wares
2000	David Wilburn Kaminski
2001	Robert Darrell Nelson
2002	Vernon Day Smith

Centennial Celebration Book Committee

Francis M. James III, co-chair

C. Douglas Maynard, co-chair

Linda T. Bell

Katherine Davis

Donna S. Garrison

Dianne Johnson

Vicki Johnson

W. Roger Poston II

Patricia L. Rice

Michael D. Sprinkle

Parks Welch